Essential Calculation Skills for Nurses, Midwives and Healthcare Practitioners

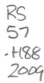

Essential Calculation Skills for Nurses, Midwives and Healthcare Practitioners

Meriel Hutton

Open University Press

Open University Press
McGraw-Hill Education
McGraw-Hill House
Shoppenhangers Road
Maidenhead
Berkshire
England
SL6 2QL

email: enquiries@openup.co.uk
world wide web: www.openup.co.uk

and Two Penn Plaza, New York, NY 10121–2289, USA

First published 2009

A catalogue record of this book is available from the British Library

ISBN 13: 978 0 335 23359 5 (PB)
ISBN 10: 0 335 23359 7 (PB)

Library of Congress Cataloging-in-Publication Data
CIP data applied for

Typeset by Graphicraft Limited, Hong Kong
Printed in UK by Bell and Bain Ltd., Glasgow

The **McGraw·Hill** Companies

Contents

CONTENTS

List of figures

Preface

This book has been written for students and healthcare practitioners who have to use and manipulate numbers in their clinical practice. The text is particularly suitable for nurses (all branches), midwives, health visitors and operating department practitioners: it is also suitable as a primer for pharmacy students and non-medical prescribers. It addresses what is currently regarded as a much required need in the delivery of care in today's health service.

Because there is a wide variation in entry level competence in numeracy, a self-assessment section allows readers to find their appropriate starting point. Thereafter, the calculations increase in the need for understanding as the chapters progress. The book is designed to be worked through sequentially at the reader's own pace.

Practice exercises are included at every stage and the answers are provided at the back of the book in Appendix E. Safety is emphasized at all times. The examples are based on the real world of modern healthcare practice and span a broad spectrum of clinical areas. I am very grateful to colleagues in clinical practice who have suggested specific scenarios within which to construct examples, particularly those at the Children's Hospital Birmingham NHS Trust and University Hospital Birmingham NHS Trust.

Above all, it is hoped that the text will be user-friendly and relevant. If those who work through the book feel more confident and are able to practise more safely, it will have succeeded in its objectives.

Meriel Hutton
July 2008

Disclaimer

It should be emphasized that this is a book on use of numbers in healthcare and not a textbook of therapeutics. While every effort has been made to check drug dosages, it is still possible that errors might occur. Furthermore, dosage schedules are continually being revised and new side-effects recognized. For these reasons, the reader should consult current drug information in the British National Formulary and product information from the manufacturers before administering any of the drugs used as examples.

Acknowledgements

I would like to thank the RPS Publishing for permission to use the information published in the British National Formulary (BNF, March 2008) throughout this book. Hospital charts and forms have been kindly provided by Royal Wolverhampton Hospitals NHS Trust, Birmingham Children's Hospital NHS Trust and University Hospital Birmingham NHS Trust for use as examples.

Grateful thanks are also due to my family for their support and encouragement and to Rachel Crookes and Jack Fray of Open University Press/McGraw-Hill who have steered me on the road to publication.

xiii

Introduction

There is a substantial background of research which suggests that the teaching and assessing of numeracy in healthcare education should be based on reality rather than the abstract teaching of mathematics. The text within this book will try to put calculations into a healthcare context. It offers different methods of calculating drug dosages and fluid prescriptions and sets out the vital steps that should be taken in order to avoid mistakes. As a book, it cannot replace real and simulated practical situations and is recommended as an additional source of help and calculation practice. In an effort to be as realistic as possible, scenarios related to the different branches of nursing are provided to allow practice of calculation skills in safety. Answers are provided to all the problems posed so that progress can be checked. Where the terms 'nursing' or 'nurses' are used, the intention is to cover nurses of all branches and also midwives, although there are specific practice examples included for the different groups. Other healthcare students such as Operating Department Practitioners may also find it a useful source for developing calculation skills.

How to use this book

To start using the book, refresh your memory of numbers and numeric functions by trying the self-assessment on p. 7. If you answer all the questions correctly with no difficulty, then you can skip the part on basic mathematical skills and go straight to where these are applied to nursing and midwifery. If you find you have difficulty in any of the calculations later on, you can always come back to the basic skills sections. If you did not get the right answers to the test, then work through the first two chapters, practise using the examples given and then try the test again. The test does not assume that you have any prior knowledge of healthcare terminology and it is also recognized that performance in the test does not necessarily predict ability to use the relevant mathematical skills in nursing and midwifery practice. However, it does include the types of calculations you will use in nursing and midwifery and so should help you decide how much help you might need in learning how to calculate medication dosages. Many universities use this sort of test at interview.

INTRODUCTION

If you have difficulty comprehending what is being asked in worded problems, this may be because of the terminology used and it is important to read these questions carefully and pick out the relevant information for the numerical calculation. This book uses healthcare terminology and common measures in healthcare from the very first chapter but is not intended as a textbook of therapeutics. If you are unfamiliar with the terms, check if they are covered in the Glossary in Appendix C. However, some people have a particular difficulty in reading and comprehending words, called **dyslexia**. The equivalent condition relating to numbers is termed **dyscalculia**. There are a number of strategies available to help individuals to overcome such problems, but these cannot be covered in the scope of this book. If you think you may have either of these conditions, *do* get yourself assessed and take advantage of the help which universities can offer. Only a small proportion of individuals with this type of learning difficulty will be unable to find adequate coping strategies. For these, however, for the safety of our patients, sadly, it is unlikely that you will be able to qualify and register as a nurse or midwife.

Each chapter of the book deals with one or more aspects of nursing care in which numbers need to be understood and calculations done. It is recommended that you work through the chapters sequentially, as the calculations become more complex as you progress through the book. Different ways of calculating are gradually introduced, so that you can choose to use what works best for you. In every chapter, where a new concept is introduced, you will find at least one worked example. Take time to work through these slowly, making sure that you understand each step of the calculation. Remember to take a break every 20 minutes or so. Tackle one section at a time and then test yourself on the practice questions. Some of these are identified as being particularly relevant to specific branches of nursing and/or to midwifery, so choose the ones which you are likely to be more familiar with first. However, most are suitable for everyone and will give you good calculation practice even if labelled as suitable for a different branch of nursing from the one which you are in. The answers to these practice exercises are given at the back of the book in Appendix E.

Abbreviations are used extensively in healthcare and can be very confusing. If ever in doubt about the correct abbreviation, always use the full word or expression so that no mistake can be made, particularly when prescribing or recording details of patient care. This text uses some medical terms and abbreviations right from the start so that practice examples are steeped in the real world of nursing. A useful list of common abbreviations can be found in Appendix A.

INTRODUCTION

This book is not designed to cover nursing practice *per se* and while the author has attempted to make examples as realistic as possible by using both drugs and dosages from a reliable source (British National Formulary, March 2008) these are included for calculation practice only and no responsibility can be taken for prescribing accuracy.

1 Numbers in Healthcare Practice

This chapter covers:

♦ The regulator's requirements

♦ Use of calculators and approximation

♦ Self-assessment

♦ Revision of numbers

Healthcare students and practitioners will come across numbers in a wide variety of situations during their work. Some of these, such as calculating drug dosages, are more obvious than others, however, all require accuracy for the safety of the patient. As a healthcare practitioner, you need to be confident that you can deal competently with any numerical situation you may come across and this book should help you to gain this confidence. If you have not already done so, read through the section in the introduction which covers how to use this book and then read on.

Numeracy requirements for nursing and midwifery

Nurses and midwives need to be able to use numbers with confidence to ensure the safety of their patients, particularly when giving medications. In January 2008, the Nursing and Midwifery Council (NMC) issued new recommendations tightening the entry requirements to programmes of preparation for registration as a nurse or midwife (NMC 2008). Universities were charged with ensuring that entrants to pre-registration education have a sufficiently good underpinning of literacy and numeracy to be able to undertake the education and practice at a minimum of diploma of higher education level. For numeracy, the specific guidance is that this includes evidence of ability to accurately manipulate numbers as applied to volume, weight and length. It also suggests that this should include skills in addition, subtraction, division, multiplication, use of decimals, fractions and percentages, and the use of a calculator.

Some universities equate this guidance regarding numeracy with a minimum entry requirement of GCSE Mathematics (grades A–C), and some ask for additional 'points' from national school examinations. Others are less prescriptive, especially where applicants are not immediate school leavers. Many universities ask applicants to pre-registration nursing and midwifery courses to do a numeracy test at interview. These tests are very varied; most seem to ask for some basic arithmetic, but also require you to interpret word problems. They may also include questions that directly relate to the problems you will have to solve in practice. These can be very difficult for someone who has never been involved with nursing care or giving medications. The diagnostic 'test' in this chapter on p. 7 is typical of the type of test you may meet at interview, but this one is deliberately *not* specific to nursing. It covers the types of arithmetic which you will need to be able to do with confidence in order to practise safely as a nurse or midwife.

As well as the slight change to entry criteria, the NMC has also added numeracy to its standards of proficiency which have to be met in order to qualify as a nurse or midwife. These are included in Essential Skills Clusters (NMC 2007a; 2007b), recently introduced to the pre-registration curricula. In the guidelines for their implementation is the requirement to test numeracy skills in relation to drug calculations at two points in the programme. For nurses, the first is at the end of the first year of the course. It is at this point that, having studied a common foundation programme, nurses will start to study their own branch of nursing in greater detail and need to demonstrate a good grounding in numeracy skills related to drug calculations.

Use of calculators

Many entry tests and nursing and midwifery educators require students to be able to calculate without resorting to a hand-held calculator. However, there are some calculations, particularly in children's and intensive care nursing which are quite complex and the use of a calculator has been demonstrated to reduce computational errors. The complexity of such calculations means that if you are using a calculator, it is vital that you understand how it works and that you are able to input the functions correctly. It is recommended that throughout this book, you attempt the calculations *without* using a calculator. However, if you work in an area where hand-held calculators are permitted, and you are in the habit of using one, first, estimate your answer and then use the calculator to do the actual calculation. If the result using the calculator is close to the estimated answer, you should be safe. If not, then start again. Never assume that the calculator is right.

Estimation/approximation

Being able to estimate or approximate the answer you are seeking is invaluable in nursing and midwifery calculations. Some errors are made by both prescribers and dispensers of medicines because they have not thought through what a sensible answer/dose would be. A quick approximation of what to expect will prevent errors of magnitude where a decimal point is misplaced and this could save a life!

In order to approximate, use your knowledge of number place and your common sense. In some cases, approximation entails rounding up or down to the nearest decimal place; in other cases the decimal fractions can be discounted. For example: when calculating the total fluid intake for an adult who is receiving up to 3000 millilitres (3 litres) of fluid over 24 hours, it would be unnecessary to include any small amounts such as the fluid content of injections, in an approximation. On the other hand, if the patient were a neonate, restricted to 12ml per hour, then an approximation *would* need to take into account even fractions of a millilitre. Always think what a sensible answer should be and if in doubt, check with someone else. Errors are made by prescribers as well as dispensers, but the accountability lies with both. You will find approximation or estimation included in the worked examples throughout the book, as well as reminders to check your answers. There is further guidance on rounding up and down in the section on decimals later in this chapter.

Test your numeracy skills

The self-assessment on p. 7 has been developed to test your understanding and skills using the basic concepts of the sort of mathematics which is needed in healthcare practice.

Attempt the self-assessment now, allowing yourself about an hour *without using a calculator*. Assess your own performance and level of understanding by checking your answers with those given at the back of the book in Appendix D. Then read on, spending time on the sections which you find less easy and testing yourself as you go.

Self-assessment

Write the following numbers in figures:

1 Fifteen thousand and thirty-four

2 One million, two hundred and six thousand, nine hundred and seven

Calculate:

3 $120 + 38 + 1395$

4 $67 + 670 + 6700$

5 $3000 - 1725$

6 $1593 - 607$

7 39×22

8 1934×9

9 $1197 \div 7$

10 $4832 \div 16$

Simplify the following fractions:

11 $\dfrac{50}{200}$

12 $\dfrac{30}{90}$

13 $\dfrac{1275}{500}$

Multiply the following fractions:

14 $\dfrac{40}{80} \times \dfrac{5}{1}$

15 $\dfrac{500}{4} \times \dfrac{15}{60}$

16 $\dfrac{7}{10} \times \dfrac{16}{1}$

17 A camera costs £45. I want to pay in 20 equal installments. How much is each payment?

18 An excursion costs £5·50 per adult and half price for children. How much will it cost for 3 adults and 5 children?

Calculate:

19 0·34 + 33 + 3·034

20 237 − 74·8

21 45·7 + 6·92 − 9·64

22 1·125 × 1000

23 0·035 × 100

24 2·2 × 3·75

25 0·4 × 43·5

26 25·5 ÷ 10

27 55·5 ÷ 100

Express as a percentage:

28 0·75

29 0·025

30 $\dfrac{9}{10}$

31 $\dfrac{4}{5}$

Express as a decimal:

32 $\dfrac{1}{4}$

33 $1\dfrac{7}{10}$

34 25%

35 80%

Express as a simple fraction:

36 0·75

37 0·05

38 20%

39 4%

Change the following metric measures:

40 500 milligrams (mg) = ? gram (g)

41 0·25 g = ? mg

42 100 millilitres (ml) = ? litres (l)

43 2mg = ? micrograms

Answers can be found at the back of the book in Appendix D.

Revision of numbers

Whole numbers

Numbers are used in lots of situations in nursing. It is important to be able to recognize number patterns and where numbers lie in order of magnitude. For example, recognizing that 1000 is 100 times bigger than 10; and 1000 times smaller than 1 million, or that 2·25 is smaller than 2·5, but bigger than 2·125. The first question in the diagnostic test relates in part to this. It is not likely that you will have to use this particular skill very often as we commonly read large numbers out digit by digit. However, there may come a time when you answer the telephone and are asked to take down some laboratory results for a patient. These results may be to do with blood cell counts, blood gas results or bacteriology counts, all of which can involve very large numbers which you need to be able to transcribe accurately. Hence, if the laboratory tells you that Mr Smith's red cell count is 5·32 million, you should be able to write it down accurately as a number.

Arranging the digits which make up any number in columns is a useful way of seeing the relationship between them and keeping them in the right order. You may remember in school having to write numbers in columns and this is a discipline that will continue to help you whatever you are trying to calculate. It is particularly useful to keep strict columns when filling out complicated fluid charts such as those used in dialysis units.

Worked example 1.1 Whole numbers

Look at the table below, where the number *five million, four hundred and twenty-five thousand, two hundred and ninety-four* is arranged in columns to show how we should write it in digits:

Millions	Thousands			Hundreds	Tens	Units
	100,000	10,000	1000			
5	4	2	5	2	9	4

Note that the thousands column can be subdivided into three columns. This is because it incorporates hundreds of thousands, tens of thousands and units of thousands.

In the UK, it is conventional when writing a number in digits, to put a comma after every three numbers, starting at the right hand side, and so *five million, four hundred and twenty-five thousand, two hundred and ninety-four* looks like this:

5,425,294

It is important to remember that using commas in this way is a convention that is not found in all countries. Many European countries do not use a comma, but leave a slight gap. Some countries use a comma to signify a decimal point, and so it is vital that you use your common sense regarding magnitude of numbers as well as just looking at what is written, especially when working with colleagues from other countries.

Worked example 1.2 More whole numbers

What about numbers which do not have a value for each column, such as: *one million, fifty-five thousand and six*?

Where there are numbers missing from the columns, just put a zero.

Millions	Thousands			Hundreds	Tens	Units
	100,000	10,000	1000			
1	0	5	5	0	0	6

Hence, *one million, fifty-five thousand and six* looks like this:

1,055,006

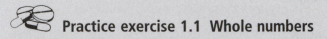

Practice exercise 1.1 Whole numbers

Write the following in numerical format:

1 One million, two hundred and thirty-four thousand, five hundred and sixty-seven

2 Five million, three hundred thousand and fifty

3 Twenty-five thousand and seven

4 One hundred and twelve thousand, six hundred

5 Eight thousand and four

Check your answers in Appendix E.

Decimals

Look at the extended table below which has columns to the right of the units column, the first of which contains a decimal point. This table can be used in the same way as we have seen for whole numbers. The difference is that these extra columns show parts or fractions of whole numbers. They are parts based on 10 and so are called *decimal fractions* or *decimals*. Fractions are explained more fully in the next section.

In the same way as we filled in the columns of the table above to write a whole number, we can use the extended table to write a number which includes a decimal fraction: *one hundred and twenty-two point six*

Hundreds	Tens	Units		Tenths	Hundreths
1	2	2	·	6	

Decimal point

The numbers to the left of the decimal point are whole numbers, while those to the right of the decimal point are parts or fractions of whole numbers. The columns indicate what fraction is signified by the number in that column. Thus:

$$\frac{6}{10} = 0{\cdot}6$$

$$\frac{6}{100} = 0{\cdot}06$$

$$\frac{6}{1000} = 0.006$$

$$\frac{6}{10000} = 0.0006$$

The decimal *nought point six* could also be written as the fraction:

$$\frac{6}{10}$$

Decimal conventions

When verbalizing decimal fractions, the fraction element is referred to as separated digits rather than a number. For example, the correct way of saying 0·55, is *nought point five five* and NOT *nought point fifty-five*.

The use of nought at either end of a decimal number is unnecessary and could be confusing. For example, 9·5 written as 09·50 could be read as a time of day, rather than a decimal fraction. The one time when it *is* not only permissible, but strongly recommended to put in the nought, is when there is no whole number, for example, 0·5. Without the nought, the decimal point may be missed and a tenfold error made. The practice of always writing a nought before the decimal point when there are no whole numbers shows the reader that the number written is less than 1.

Decimal places and rounding numbers

Placement of the decimal point is obviously very important as moving it one place in either direction alters the value of the number by a factor of 10. This is a common source of drug error and can prove fatal if 10 times a dose is given by mistake because of a misplaced decimal point or, as shown above, a missed decimal point.

The columns to the right of the decimal point are counted as 'decimal places'. The number 122·65 has two decimal places.

Rounding of decimals is done to an expressed number of decimal places. If the required number is to have fewer decimal places than the number we have, then we round it up or down in the following way:

♦ If the digit directly to the right of the last decimal place required is less than 5, the last required digit is not altered.

♦ If the digit directly to the right of the last decimal place required is 5 or larger, then the last required digit is increased by one.

Worked example 1.3 Rounding decimals

5·463 rounded to two decimal places would be 5·46.

5·468 rounded to two decimal places would be 5·47.

As you can see from the diagram:

5·463 is closer to 5·460 than to 5·470.

5·468 is closer to 5·470 than it is to 5·460.

```
5·470
  9
  8
  7
  6
  5
  4
  3
  2
  1
5·460
```

Note that we do not need to show the final nought when writing the number:

5·460 is written as 5·46.

5·470 is written as 5·47.

The same convention is applied if we need to round a decimal to the nearest whole number:

5·46 would round down to 5.

5·5 would round up to 6.

An example in healthcare where it might be necessary to round a decimal fraction to a whole number is in the instance of calculating the rate of an intravenous infusion for use with a volumetric pump. It may be necessary to round the decimal to the nearest whole number, as some devices which deliver intravenous fluids can only be programmed to the nearest millilitre per hour or per minute. Similarly, some calculations of drug dosage may result in values that are so small as to be meaningless for the kinds of measurements used. For example, a calculation which results in 1·86 tablets to be administered is meaningless. A tablet cannot practically be divided into $\frac{86}{100}$ and so in this case it would be sensible to round it up the decimal fraction and give two tablets.

13

Practice exercise 1.2 Rounding decimals

Round to one decimal place:

1 245·37   2 12·146

3 30·098   4 8·55

Round to two decimal places:

5 13·294   6 0·295

7 50·899   8 1·845

Round to the nearest whole number:

9 100·49   10 6·51

Check your answers in Appendix E.

Fractions

As we saw above, in the same way as we filled in columns to write a whole number, we can use the extended table to write a number which includes a decimal. Using decimals is a particular way of expressing parts of a number. Parts of a number may also be written as *fractions*:

One hundred and twenty-two point six

Hundreds	Tens	Units		Tenths
1	2	2	·	6

Decimal point

By arranging this number in the columns we can see that 'point six' really means six-tenths. This can be written as 6/10 or $\frac{6}{10}$ and when written like this, is called a fraction.

A fraction indicates that division is occurring. The top number (**numerator**) represents the original number of parts; the bottom number (**denominator**) represents the number which is doing the dividing; and the line between them indicates division. For example: $\frac{1}{2}$ an hour is equal to 1 of the parts when an hour is divided into two equal parts and $\frac{3}{4}$ of an hour is equal to 3 of the parts, when an hour is divided into 4 equal parts. Note that the unit of measurement written next to a fraction refers to the numerator only. Thus $\frac{1}{2}$ an hour is one hour divided by two.

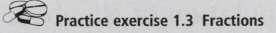 **Practice exercise 1.3 Fractions**

Express the following decimal fractions as fractions or mixed numbers:

1 0·5

2 10·7

3 1·06

4 0·35

5 0·109

Check your answers in Appendix E.

Fractions can be made up of any number divided by another. If the numerator is bigger than the denominator, it is called a **top-heavy fraction** and simplifying it may result in a **mixed number**, that is a whole number and a fraction.

Thus, $3/2 = 1\frac{1}{2}$.

Now that you have revised whole numbers, decimals and fractions, take a break before moving on to the next chapter. This will cover how these numbers are used in arithmetic and give examples of applications to everyday tasks in nursing and midwifery.

15

References

NMC (2007a) Introduction of Essential Skills Clusters for pre-registration nursing programmes. NMC Circular 07/2007. Available at: http://www.nmc-uk.org/aArticle.aspx?articleID=27908Keyword=circulars

NMC (2007b) Introduction of Essential Skills Clusters for pre-registration midwifery programmes. NMC Circular 23/2007. Available at: http://www.nmc-uk.org/aArticle.aspx?articleID=27908Keyword=circulars

NMC (2008) Evidence of literacy and numeracy required for entry to pre-registration nursing and midwifery programmes. NMC Circular 03/2008.

2 Manipulation of Numbers in Healthcare Practice

This chapter covers:

- **Whole numbers**: addition, subtraction, multiplication and division
- **Decimals**: addition, subtraction, multiplication and division
- **Fractions**: addition, subtraction, multiplication and division
- **Equations**
- **Percentage, ratio and proportion**

Basic mathematical operations

Numbers in nursing calculations need to be manipulated by using the basic arithmetic operations outlined below:

- **Addition** is the process of putting numbers together or combining them to find their *sum*.
- **Subtraction** is the opposite of addition, resulting in their *difference*.
- **Multiplication** is repeated addition. The number is added to itself a specific number of times resulting in the *product*.
- **Division** is the process of separating an amount into an equal number of parts. The result is the *quotient*.

Addition and subtraction are arithmetical processes which are used extensively in nursing and midwifery. Their most common use is probably in fluid balance charts (FBC). Whole number addition and subtraction are taught in schools from an early age and will not be covered here. However, it is recommended that the discipline of keeping numbers in columns is followed when you enter data onto charts such as the FBC. You will need to use the skills of addition and subtraction in many types of calculations covered by this book.

Multiplication

Multiplication is really a fast way of adding. A number added to itself a specific number of times is the same as multiplying it by that number. As multiplication as a process does not often cause difficulties with calculation, its use with whole numbers will not be covered here other than as a reminder.

Several words and symbols are used to indicate multiplication:

Word or symbol	Example
of	Two *of* those 5 millilitre (ml) teaspoons is 10ml
times	Two *times* a 5ml teaspoonful is 10ml
×	2 × 5ml = 10ml
*	2*5ml = 10ml
( )( )	(2)(5ml) = 10ml

Multiplying any number by 1 does not change the number: $5 \times 1 = 5$.

Try Practice exercise 2.1 by solving the multiplication calculations in the written problems.

Practice exercise 2.1 Multiplication of whole numbers

1 A service user has to take 6 tablets per day. How many will they take in a week?

2 If a patient is prescribed 15mls every hour, how much will they have had in 8 hours?

3 How many hours will a nurse have worked after 23 12-hour shifts?

Check your answers in Appendix E.

Division

Division is another matter and many students find this difficult. Most have been used to using a hand-held calculator and have forgotten how to divide from first principles. For this reason we will go over the process of both short and long division of whole numbers at this point to refresh your memory.

Division is the process of separating something into equal parts. Thus, a daily total of 50 milligrams (mg) of medicine, to be taken in equal amounts twice a day means taking

50 ÷ 2 = 25mg per dose

Any number can be divided by 1 without changing its value. Thus, a daily amount of 50mg taken once a day would be

50 ÷ 1 = 50mg per dose

Several words and symbols are used to indicate division.

Word or symbol	Example
for	50mg *for* two doses = 25mg
/	50mg/2 doses = 25mg
—	$\dfrac{50mg}{2\ doses}$ = 25mg per dose
÷	50mg ÷ 2 doses = 25mg per dose
$\overline{)}$	$2\overline{)50}$ = 25

Some division you will be able to do easily in your head. For example, if there are 6 chocolates left in the box and 3 people who want them, how many can they have each?

6 ÷ 3 = 2

If you cannot do the division in your head, then there are two ways of setting out the process to make it easier. One is called **short division** and the other **long division**.

Short division is used to find how many times a number will go into another when the *divisor*, or the number doing the dividing, is small, but the *dividend*, or the number being divided, is relatively large.

Worked example 2.1 Short division (i)

You are part of a lottery syndicate of 6 colleagues. Your numbers come up and you win £372 to share between you. How much should each member get? In other words, you need to divide 372 into 6 equal parts.

To divide 372 by 6, follow the steps below:

$$6\overline{)3\ 7\ 2}$$

First, it is vital to get the divisor (6) and the dividend (372) in the correct place when setting up the division calculation. Once set up, we then try dividing number by number:

$$6\ \ 2$$
$$6\overline{)3\ {}^3 7\ {}^1 2}$$

6 into 3 'won't go' and so we leave a space above the 3 and try 6 into 37. From multiplication tables, we know that 6×6 is 36 and so we can put 6 above the 7.

The 1 left over from dividing 6 into 37 is carried forward to make 12 the next dividend. 6 into 12 goes exactly twice and so we put a 2 above the 12.

And so, $372 \div 6 = 62$.

We can check that this is correct by multiplying back up:

$6 \times 62 = 372$

Worked example 2.2 Short division (ii)

Divide 516 by 5:

$$5\,\overline{|\,5\ 1\ 6}$$

Follow the same steps as in Worked example 2.1:

$$\begin{array}{r} 1\ 0\ 3 \\ 5\,\overline{|\,5\ 1\ {}^16} \\ \text{Remainder 1} \end{array}$$

5 into 5 goes once, so we put a 1 over the 5. As there is nothing over, we then try 5 into the next digit, 1.

5 will not go into 1, so put a nought above the 1 and carry it forward to make the next number 16.

5 goes into 16 three times ($5 \times 3 = 15$) with 1 left over. So we put a 3 over the 16 and comment that there is 1 remaining.

And so, $516 \div 5 = 103$ remainder 1.

In this example the division is not exact and there is 1 left over. We will deal with remainders later on in this chapter.

Long division is used when you do not know the multiplication table relating to the divisor. It is just the same as short division but elongates the working so that the space under the bar does not get too cramped with the large numbers left over at each stage.

Worked example 2.3 Long division

You move to a different hospital and join another lottery syndicate which is made up of all the theatre staff, a total of 63 people. Again your numbers come up and the syndicate wins a total of £34,524. We need to divide 34,524 into 63 equal parts, but we don't know the 63 times table.

First, set up the division as shown for short division:

$$63\,\overline{|\,3\ 4\ 5\ 2\ 4}$$

Now divide. Long division is the same process as short division except that because the numbers concerned are bigger, your working is set out underneath the 'sum' instead of using superscript. By writing down the result of multiplying the divisor by a suitable number, the subtraction sum, which in short division you did in your head, in set out for you and the remainder to carry forward is provided automatically. Carefully follow the explanation to the left of the long-division sum set out below.

We can see that 63 will not go into 3 or 34, so we put a nought or zero above those numbers at this point or we can leave a space. The 34 is now 'carried forward' to make the next number we need to look at, which is 345. As we don't know the 63 times table, we have to make an estimate for how many times 63 will go into 345. By rounding the numbers, we can make an educated guess that it will be about 5, since $60 \times 5 = 300$. We write 5 on the top line next to the zeros and write the

```
      0 0 5 4 8
63 │ 3 4 5 2 4
     3 1 5
     ──────
     3 0 2
     2 5 2
     ──────
       5 0 4
       5 0 4
       ──────
       0 0 0
```

product of 5×63 (315) under the 345. We subtract 315 from 345 to get a remainder of 30. We then bring down the next number (2) from the original dividend, keeping it directly under where it comes from and start dividing again. This time we are looking for how many times 63 will go into 302. We can see that 5 times is too big and so we try 4 times. The 4 goes on the top line over the 2. The product of 4×63 is 252 which we write underneath the 302 and subtract to get the remainder. This time it is 50. When we bring down the last remaining number from the original dividend in the same way as before, we get 504. This time 63 will go 8 times and so we put an 8 on the top line and when we subtract the product of 8×63 (504) from 504 we are left with nothing and our working is complete.

And so, £34,524 ÷ 63 = £548

Each member of the syndicate should receive £548.

Practice exercise 2.2 Division of whole numbers

1 If a patient is to have a total of 450mg of a drug in 3 divided doses, how many milligrams in each dose? (450 ÷ 3)

2 An intravenous infusion of 1000ml is prescribed to last 5 hours. How much fluid should be delivered each hour? (1000 ÷ 5)

3 A delivery of 1500 new pillows has arrived at the hospital. If there are 23 wards, how many should go to each ward? How many will remain? (1500 ÷ 23)

4 How much will you be able to afford on rent each week if you have budgeted £7,800 per year? (7800 ÷ 52)

Check your answers in Appendix E.

We have just practised using the basic arithmetic functions with whole numbers. Now let's see how these skills transfer to decimals and fractions.

Addition and subtraction of decimals

Adding and subtracting decimals are not difficult if you keep to the discipline of lining up the decimal points as in Worked example 2.4.

Worked example 2.4 Addition of decimals

Add 2·5 to 125·25 like this:

$$
\begin{array}{r}
2 \cdot 5 \\
1\ 2\ 5 \cdot 2\ 5\ + \\
\hline
1\ 2\ 7 \cdot 7\ 5
\end{array}
$$

If it makes it easier, you can add zeros beyond the digits on either side of the decimal point without changing the value but remember that they should not appear in the final answer.

$$
\begin{array}{r}
0\ 0\ 2 \cdot 5\ 0 \\
1\ 2\ 5 \cdot 2\ 5\ + \\
\hline
1\ 2\ 7 \cdot 7\ 5
\end{array}
$$

Worked example 2.5 Subtraction of decimals

Do subtraction the same way, for example, to subtract 65·75 from 124·8:

$$
\begin{array}{r}
1\ 2\ 4\ \cdot\ 8\ 0 \\
0\ 6\ 5\ \cdot\ 7\ 5\ - \\
\hline
0\ 5\ 9\ \cdot\ 0\ 5
\end{array}
$$

It is always good practice to approximate your answer before doing the calculation and to cross-check afterwards. In addition of two numbers, you can check by subtracting one of them from your answer, which should give you the other number. So, in the examples above, if you subtract 2·5 from 127·75, you get 125·25. This confirms that you have added them correctly. Similarly, after subtracting one number from another, by adding one of the original numbers to your answer, you will get the other original number.

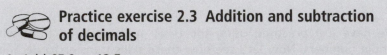

Practice exercise 2.3 Addition and subtraction of decimals

1 Add 65·9 to 12·5.

2 Subtract 125·5 from 180.

3 Add 5·025 to 20·75.

4 Subtract 34·45 from 118·9.

5 Add 90, 180, 2·75, 1·6.

Check your answers using estimation and by cross-checking as suggested above before turning to the answers in Appendix E.

Multiplying decimals

When multiplying decimals by 10 or multiples of 10, the decimal point can be moved to the right, as many spaces as there are noughts after the multiplier, resulting in a bigger number.

Remember that multiplying is just a fast way of adding, for example, we can check this by trying $6·5 \times 10$. Multiplying 6·5 by 10 is the same as adding 10 lots of 6 to 10 lots of 0·5:

$(10 \times 6) + (10 \times 0·5)$

$= 60 + 5$

$= 65$

which is what we would have got if we had simply moved the decimal point one place to the right: $6·5 \rightarrow 65$.

Mistakes are made in nursing calculations when the decimal point is wrongly placed. A decimal point can be moved only when multiplying or dividing by 10 or multiples of 10. Always do an estimate.

Worked example 2.6 Multiplying decimals (i)

Multiply 10×1.25. Estimate either by looking at it as an addition (10 lots of 1 plus 10 lots of 0.25) or by rounding the numbers to the nearest whole number $10 \times 1 = 10$. Either way, our answer should be in the magnitude of 10.

Move the decimal place *one* space to the right as there is one nought in 10:

$$10 \times 1.25 = 12.5$$

And check this against our estimate. The actual answer of 12.5 is the same magnitude as our estimate of 10. Had our answer been 125 or 1.25, we would know immediately that the decimal point was in the wrong place.

Worked example 2.7 Multiplying decimals (ii)

Multiply 1000×0.52. Estimate by rounding the numbers. 0.5 is equal to a half and half of 1000 is 500, so our answer should be about 500.

Now multiply by 1000 by moving the decimal place *three* spaces to the right:

$$1000 \times 0.52 = 520$$

which is close to our estimate.

Decimal numbers can be multiplied by whole numbers or by decimals in the same way as whole numbers are multiplied together, with the additional step of making sure that the same number of digits lies to the right of the decimal point in the answer as there were in both the original numbers.

Worked example 2.8 Multiplying decimals (iii)

A mother tells you she is giving her baby a 6·5oz bottle. What is this amount in millilitres (ml)? You know that 1 fluid ounce is equal to 28·4ml and so the calculation will be 6.5×28.4.

Do a rough estimation by rounding the numbers to the nearest whole number as this will help you place the decimal point correctly:

$7 \times 28 = 196$

Now set up the multiplication sum:

On this row we are multiplying the top row by 0·5.
On this row we are multiplying the top row by 6.
Here we have added them together.

$$
\begin{array}{r}
2\ 8\ \cdot\ 4 \\
6\ \cdot\ 5 \quad \times \\
\hline
1\ 4\ \cdot\ 2\ 0 \\
1\ 7\ 0\ \cdot\ 4\ 0 \\
\hline
1\ 8\ 4\ \cdot\ 6\ 0
\end{array}
$$

Both original numbers have *one* number following the decimal point and so the answer needs *two* numbers following the decimal point.

$28·4 \times 6·5 = 184·60$

Check this against the estimate. Remember that having completed our calculation, we can drop the final nought to the right of the decimal point without changing the value of our answer. Thus, our final answer is 184·6ml.

 Practice exercise 2.4 Multiplying decimals

1 $2·75 \times 10$

2 $1·25 \times 1000$

3 $345·7 \times 1·2$

4 $28·4 \times 24$

5 $200 \times 0·075$

Check your answers in Appendix E.

Dividing decimals

Dividing decimals by 10 or multiples of 10 is just the same as multiplying them except that the decimal point moves to the left and the number becomes smaller.

Dividing decimals by decimals is done by changing the divisor (the number doing the dividing) into a whole number and then using the process of long or short division keeping the decimal point in the same place for the answer.

Worked example 2.9 Dividing decimals (i)

A baby weighs 8·14lb and you want to know what this is in kilograms. There are 2·2lb in 1kg and so we need to divide 8·14 by 2·2 to convert from pounds to kilograms.

Estimate an answer first.

We can get a rough estimate by remembering that the same weight will be a higher number of pounds (lb) than it is kilograms (kg).

By rounding the numbers, we get 8 ÷ 2 = 4, and so our answer should be approximately 4.

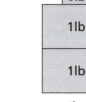

Now calculate. As we saw earlier, a number divided by another can be written 10/2, meaning 10 divided by 2. If we multiply both these numbers by the same number, the value of the answer will not change:

Just as $\dfrac{10}{2} = 5$, $\dfrac{10 \times 4}{2 \times 4}$ or $\dfrac{40}{8} = 5$

So, to change the decimal divisor of our problem (2·2) to a whole number, the easiest thing is to multiply by 10 to get 22. We then have to do the same thing to the dividend (8·14) and we get 81·4.

So 8·14 ÷ 2·2 is the same as 81·4 ÷ 22.

We can now use long division as we did using whole numbers, but keeping the decimal point in the same place:

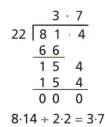

8·14 ÷ 2·2 = 3·7

By checking against the estimate, we can see that the decimal point is in the right place and our answer is 3·7kg.

Worked example 2.10 Dividing decimals (ii)

The shifts at your hospital last 7·5 hours each. How many shifts would you need to do to make up 1222 practice hours?

First, estimate using numbers to which you can easily relate:

e.g. $1400 \div 7 = 200$

Next change the decimal divisor into a whole number and change the dividend accordingly, i.e. multiply both by 10.

Now proceed with long division:

There comes a point with long division where the common sense of what you are doing should tell you to stop. In this instance we are looking for a number of shifts and so we want a whole number. The answer we have reached (so far), if rounded up to the next whole number will give us an answer of 163 and this is in the same area of magnitude as our estimate. In the same way we can correct an answer to any number of decimal places by rounding up where the next number is 5 or

```
                     1 6 2 · 9
          75  1 2 2 2 0 · 0
              7 5
              4 7 2
              4 5 0
                2 2 0
                1 5 0
                  7 0  0
                  6 7  5
                    2  5
```

above. Note that the decimal place did not need to be there when we began our division, but was put in when we ran out of numbers to bring down. In exactly the same way the remainder in a division of whole numbers can be transformed into a decimal fraction.

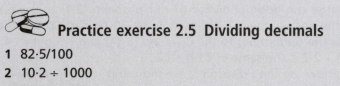

Practice exercise 2.5 Dividing decimals

1 82·5/100

2 10·2 ÷ 1000

3 58·79 ÷ 2·2 *(correct to 1 decimal place)*

4 653·2 ÷ 28·4

5 12·5/0·5

Check your answers in Appendix E.

Changing decimals to fractions

You may recognize *point two five* (written 0·25) as a commonly used decimal fraction, equivalent to $\frac{1}{4}$. How is 0·25 the same as $\frac{1}{4}$?

From the number columns used in Chapter 1 on pp. 11–12, we know that 0·25 is the same as 25 hundredths or 25/100. To turn 25 hundredths into quarters, we need to simplify or cancel down the fraction to reduce it to its simplest form.

Simplifying fractions or cancelling down

Sometimes the numbers in the numerator and the denominator are related to each other so that the fraction can be simplified to remain a fraction but without changing its value. For example, we could express $\frac{1}{2}$ hour as $\frac{2}{4}$ hour. This would mean the same, but it is conventional to write a fraction in its simplest form, in this case, $\frac{1}{2}$.

To simplify fractions, unless you are very confident of the factors which make up the numbers you are dealing with, start by dividing both the numerator (top) and denominator (bottom) of the fraction by the biggest number which you can see will go into both of them exactly. In our example, we can divide both the top and bottom of the fraction $\frac{2}{4}$ by 2 and this gives us $\frac{1}{2}$. Whatever you do to the top, you must also do to the bottom so that the value of the fraction does not change. This process is referred to as cancelling down.

Worked example 2.11 Simplifying fractions or cancelling down

Returning to the task of expressing 0·25 as a fraction, we need to simplify 25/100:

$$\frac{25}{100} = \frac{\overset{5}{\cancel{25}}}{\underset{20}{\cancel{100}}} = \frac{5}{20} \qquad \text{And again} \qquad \frac{\overset{1}{\cancel{5}}}{\underset{4}{\cancel{20}}} = \frac{1}{4}$$

First, we divided both top and bottom by 5. The fraction is still not as simple as it could be, so we can divide again by 5 and reach our goal of $\frac{1}{4}$.

It is useful to recognize equivalent fractions and decimals which you may come across in healthcare. The shaded areas in the diagrams below show some common equivalents.

The shaded area is half of each shape and so all the fractions below are equivalent to half or 0·5.

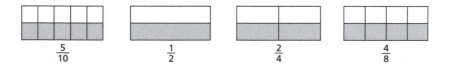

$$\frac{5}{10} \qquad\qquad \frac{1}{2} \qquad\qquad \frac{2}{4} \qquad\qquad \frac{4}{8}$$

In the same way, the fractions below are equivalent to 0·25.

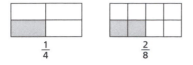

$\frac{1}{4}$ $\qquad$ $\frac{2}{8}$

Changing fractions to decimals

This is simply a matter of dividing in the way we have already practised:

$\frac{1}{4}$ = 1 divided by 4

$$4\overline{)1 \cdot 0\ 0}$$

$$\begin{array}{r} 0 \cdot\ 2\ \ 5 \\ 4\overline{)1 \cdot\ {}^{1}0\ {}^{2}0} \end{array}$$

= 0·25

  Practice exercise 2.6 Changing decimals to fractions and fractions to decimals

Write down the following numbers in figures, using decimals or fractions where asked:

1 Forty and a quarter (as a decimal).
2 Simplify 56/140 and express as a fraction.
3 Simplify 147/63 and express as a mixed number.
4 What is 0·125 as a simplified fraction?
5 Change 32/50 to a decimal.
6 What fraction of the whole figure is the shaded area?

7 What is this as a decimal?

Check your answers in Appendix E.

Addition and subtraction of fractions

It is not often in nursing that you will need this skill, but you do need to be aware of the process and we'll use a simple example to illustrate it:

$$\frac{1}{2} + \frac{1}{4} = \frac{3}{4}$$

In order to do the sum, we had to change the fractions so that they had the same denominator. This is the opposite of cancelling down and requires us to find the lowest number that will allow us to change both fractions (if necessary) to have the same denominator. This is called the *lowest common denominator*. In this example, we can easily change the $\frac{1}{2}$ to quarters by multiplying both top and bottom by 2 (remember that as long as we do the same to both top and bottom, the fraction keeps the same value):

$$\frac{1}{2} \times \frac{2}{2} = \frac{2}{4}$$

Now that we have both fractions with the same denominator, we can add (or subtract as the case may be) across the numerators:

$$\frac{2}{4} + \frac{1}{4} = \frac{2+1}{4} = \frac{3}{4}$$

Look back at the columns on p. 11 in Chapter 1 where we arranged 122·6. This explains how 0·25, as 2 tenths and 5 hundredths, was then referred to as 25 hundredths. By multiplying both top and bottom of the two tenths fraction, we get twenty hundredths and can then add the two fractions:

$$\frac{2}{10} + \frac{5}{100} = \frac{20}{100} + \frac{5}{100} = \frac{20+5}{100} = \frac{25}{100}$$

We then simplified this by cancelling down to finish with $\frac{1}{4}$.

> ### Practice exercise 2.7 Addition and subtraction of fractions
>
> 1 Add $\frac{3}{8} + \frac{3}{4}$
>
> 2 Subtract $\frac{3}{4} - \frac{2}{3}$
>
> 3 Add $\frac{1}{2} + \frac{2}{3}$
>
> 4 Subtract $\frac{5}{6} - \frac{1}{4}$
>
> *Check your answers in Appendix E.*

Multiplying and dividing fractions

This is something that you will have to do a lot if you use the formula for drug dosage calculation (see Chapter 4, p. 66) and also when calculating drip rates for intravenous infusions or intragastric feeds in neonates. This section will explain the process in principle, using simple examples.

Worked example 2.12 Multiplying fractions

The amount of fluid in half a cup which holds 180 millilitres (ml), is half *of* 180, which is 90. Follow the process above: *of* is turned into × and 180 is shown as $\frac{180}{1}$:

$$\frac{1}{2} \times \frac{180}{1} = \frac{180}{2}$$

To multiply the fractions, multiply across the top row (numerators) to get 180 and multiply across the bottom row (denominators) to get 2.

The calculation could be simplified by cancelling down the original fractions. Where denominator and numerator can be divided exactly by the same number, we can simplify. This is also possible across a multiplication sign as the value of the final fraction will not be altered.

Thus:

$$\frac{1}{2} \times \frac{180}{1} = \frac{1}{\overset{}{\underset{1}{2}}} \times \frac{\overset{90}{\cancel{180}}}{1}$$

$$= 90$$

Dividing fractions is not often required in the calculations nurses have to make. The process is the same as multiplication of fractions except that the second fraction must be turned the other way up.

Look at the example. We could say that to get half of 180, we need to divide by 2. This is exactly the same as multiplying by a half:

$$\frac{180}{1} \div \frac{2}{1} = \frac{180}{1} \times \frac{1}{2}$$

$$= 90$$

Practice exercise 2.8 Multiplying and dividing fractions

Calculate the following and simplify where appropriate:

1 $\dfrac{3}{4} \times \dfrac{1}{5}$

2 $\dfrac{1}{2}$ of $\dfrac{3}{5}$

3 $\dfrac{1}{3} \times \dfrac{3}{5}$

4 $\dfrac{6}{8} \div 2$

5 $\dfrac{5}{14} / \dfrac{2}{7}$

Check your answers in Appendix E.

Equations

We have been using equations already. Every time we use an equals sign, we are effectively displaying an equation where one side equals the other. The golden rule of equations is that whatever you do to one side, you must do to the other, in order to keep the balance.

In an equation, we might have an unknown value on one side. For example, when calculating how fast an intravenous infusion is to run, we want to know its rate. Rate is a measurement of something happening over time. For example, the rate of travel by car is expressed in miles per hour using the formula below:

$$Rate = \frac{Distance}{Time}$$

If a car travels 60 miles in 2 hours, its rate is

$$\frac{60}{2} = 30 \text{ miles per hour}$$

Similarly we can use the following formula for the rate of an intravenous infusion:

$$Rate = \frac{Volume}{Time}$$

The prescription for the infusion will tell us the volume and the time in which it is to be delivered, but the rate is what we do not know and want to work out.

Worked example 2.13 Simple equations

For an infusion of 500ml to be delivered in 6 hours, the rate will be:

$$Rate = \frac{Volume}{Time}$$

$$Rate = \frac{500}{6} \text{ ml per hour}$$

Set up the short division calculation:

$$6 \overline{)\ 500}$$

$$\begin{array}{c} 8\ \ 3\ \cdot\ \ 3\ \ 3 \\ \hline 6\ \overline{)\ 5\ \ ^50\ \ ^20\ \cdot\ \ ^20\ \ ^20} \end{array}$$

$$= 83 \cdot 333 \text{ml per hour}$$

So the infusion should be delivered at 83·333ml per hour. The decimal fraction above could be rounded down to 83ml per hour depending on the settings of the delivery device.

Another use of the equation is if we knew at what rate the fluid was being delivered and wanted to know what time the amount in the container would be finished. Let us say that there is 100ml left in the bottle and the rate is set at 50ml per hour. We can use the same equation:

$$Rate = \frac{Volume}{Time} \quad \text{or} \quad r = \frac{v}{t}$$

but this time we can substitute values for rate and volume:

$$50 = \frac{100}{t}$$

Time (t) is what we want to find out and it's on the bottom of the fraction. What do we need to do to get *t* in the right position to give us our answer?

Remember that whatever we do to one side of the equation, we can do to the other without changing the value. So, multiply both sides by the unknown factor (*t*) to get it where we want it.

This will give us:

$$50 \times t = \frac{100}{t} \times \frac{t}{1}$$

We can cancel out the two *t*s on the right side of the equation and are left with:

$$50 \times t = 100$$

In order to get *t* on its own, this time we need to divide both sides of the equation by 50:

$$\frac{50 \times t}{50} = \frac{100}{50}$$

If we cancel the two 50s on the left, we now have a value for *t*:

$$t = \frac{100}{50} = 2 \text{ hours}$$

so we can say that the fluid will run out in 2 hours.

Practice exercise 2.9 Solving simple equations

Find the value of the letter in each of these equations correct to one decimal place:

1 $r = \dfrac{1000}{6}$

2 $125 = \dfrac{500}{t}$

3 $125 = \dfrac{v}{8}$

Check your answers in Appendix E.

Percentages (%), ratios and proportions

Percentages are usually seen in healthcare practice on labelling of drugs or intravenous fluids and it is seldom required to factor them into the calculation itself. However, it is important to understand what is meant by percentage (%) so that you can interpret dosages if necessary. Per cent literally means per 100, and in healthcare, percentage solutions usually refer to grams of solid dissolved in 100ml of solution.

Sometimes drugs are packaged as a *ratio* or *proportion*, such as 1:1000 adrenaline. As manipulation of the numbers involved in such preparations is neither easy nor particularly common, calculations related to percentages, ratios and proportions are dealt with in Chapter 8.

The next chapter will look at the use of numbers associated with common measurements in nursing and midwifery.

3 Common Measurements in Healthcare Practice

Money management

Since 1971, the UK has used a metric system for currency, which makes keeping accounts much easier. Many nurses, particularly those working in community and residential care homes, have to deal with money as part of their role, whether it is keeping track of clients' own cash when shopping or taking into account the cost of individual drugs when prescribing medication. The calculations concerned are not difficult but a robust system of keeping account of money gives clarity to patients/clients and their relatives and may protect you from being accused of dishonesty. Using a simple credit/debit account is useful for record keeping and can be used with a running total (account style 1) or totted up at the end of the week (account style 2) in Worked example 3.1.

Decimal coinage is treated in the same way as decimal fractions and just as with addition and subtraction, keeping figures in columns is recommended. Alternatively, printed accounts note books are available.

Worked example 3.1 Weekly accounts

The care home where you work arranges for its residents to sell their craftwork through a retail outlet. Mrs Jones wishes to know how her funds are being accounted for and so you help her to set up a week per page record as illustrated below. This could equally be done for a monthly record depending on the frequency of transactions.

Notice how in account style 1 the balance is calculated each time there is an entry by adding figures in rows from the credit (paid in) column and subtracting from the debit (spent) column. At the end of December, she had £314·60 in her account.

Account style 1

Date	Item	Credit				Debit				Running Balance				
		£		p		£		p		£			p	
BALANCE brought forward from previous week, 31/12										3	1	4	6	0
3/1	Pension	8	7	9	8					4	0	2	5	8
4/1	Sale of work	1	2	4	0					4	1	4	9	8
5/1	Coffees						6	5	0	4	0	8	4	8
5/1	Papers						6	2	7	4	0	2	2	1
6/1	BALANCE to take forward to following week									4	0	2	2	1

In the second example, the balance is calculated at the end of the week by adding up the columns and then subtracting the total debit from the total credit.

Account style 2

Date	Item	Credit				Debit				Balance				
		£		p		£		p		£			p	
31/12	BALANCE brought forward									3	1	4	6	0
3/1	Pension	8	7	9	8									
4/1	Sale of work	1	2	4	0									
5/1	Coffees						6	5	0					
5/1	Papers						6	2	7					
Week's total		1	0	0	3	8	1	2	7	7		8	7	6	1
6/1	BALANCE to take forward									4	0	2	2	1

Practice exercise 3.1 Money management (particularly suitable for Learning Disability and Mental Health nursing)

To help you answer the questions below, devise a balance sheet which clearly shows income and expenditure for the week described.

William Wills is a client with a learning disability who lives in a community home and wants to go shopping for some personal items. He has £27·60 in his purse. On Monday, a group of clients are taken to the local shopping centre by the nursing staff. When he returns to the home, William claims that he has been robbed. He has purchased the following items:

   3 pairs of socks @ £1·25 per pair

   A pack of 3 handkerchiefs for £1·99

   A jumper priced £8·48

1 How much did William spend?

2 How much change should he have in his purse?

William then finds 50 pence in his pocket and is satisfied that he has not been cheated.

3 How much was in William's purse when he thought he had been robbed?

On Sunday, it is William's birthday and his relatives visit to give him a number of cheques. Aunt Jane's is for £20, cousin Luke gives him £35 and Uncle Reg gives him £50. His nephew Tom gives him £6.35 cash that he has earned doing odd jobs at home and little Rosie gives him her week's pocket money of 75 pence.

4 How much did he receive all together?

William puts £1.50 into the vending machine to buy chocolate bars, which he shares with the children.

5 Assuming that he has not spent any other money since the outing, how much should he now have in total?

Check your answers in Appendix E.

Time and the 24-hour clock

In hospitals the 24-hour clock is usually, but not always, used to record time. This can be confusing and as with all numerical dealings, you must use common sense to interpret what you see.

Times using the 24-hour clock should be written as follows:

8 am = 08.00 hrs

12 midday = 12.00 hrs

8 pm = 20.00 hrs

12 midnight = 00.00 hrs

When calculating times, although they look like decimal numbers, remember *that they are not* and that there are 60 minutes in an hour. Hence, 14.59 is one minute to three in the afternoon.

Worked example 3.2 The 24-hour clock

You are due to attend an interview in the nearby city at 09.30 hrs. The train service from your local station is reliable and it takes 43 minutes to reach the city. The trains are very punctual, arriving on the hour and then at 20-minute intervals, but you can't find the timetable with arrival times, and the website is down. The letter inviting you to interview states that the venue is a 5-minute walk from the station. You want to allow an additional 10 minutes to find the place and get composed before the interview. What train do you need to catch?

The easiest way is to work backwards from the time you want to arrive. You want to arrive 10 minutes before 09.30. Easy, that's 09.20.

The walk from the station is 5 minutes and so you need to catch a train which arrives before 5 minutes prior to 09.20. Easy again, that means a train that gets in by 09.15.

If the journey from your local station takes 43 minutes, which train will get you there by 09.15?

09.15 minus 43 minutes

Remember that these are not decimal fractions but times based on 60 minutes in an hour. So when we subtract, we need to bear that in mind.

To make the subtraction easier, we can consider	8 . 7 5 hrs
9 hours and 15 minutes as equivalent to 8 hours	. 4 3
and 75 minutes.	8 . 3 2

So now you know that you will need to catch a train before 08.32. As they leave at 20-minute intervals past the hour, you will be able to catch the 08.20 and arrive in good time.

COMMON MEASUREMENTS IN HEALTHCARE PRACTICE

Practice exercise 3.2 Time (suitable for all)

1 Your shift begins at 07.30 and you are expected to work until 15.00 with an hour off for lunch. How long is the shift?

2 Baby James is to be given a feed every 3 hours. When you look at his record card you note that he was last fed at 22.40 hrs. What time is his next feed due?

3 You are told at handover that Mr Brown's intravenous infusion is due through at 14.30. If the fluid was prescribed to be delivered over 8 hours, what time was it put up?

4 Angie is an anorexic teenager who has negotiated to eat a meal every $4\frac{1}{2}$ hours during the day. She had breakfast at 07.45. What time should she have lunch?

5 Bill has learning difficulties and can become very distressed if his daily routine is upset. He likes to watch a TV programme which starts at 17.20. If the bus journey from the day centre to his home is 25 minutes and it takes him 6 minutes to get settled in front of the TV, what is the latest time he must leave in order to get him home in time for his programme?

Check your answers in Appendix E.

39

Metric units

In 1975, the healthcare profession in UK discarded the use of Imperial units such as ounces, inches, and pints in favour of a metric system based on the Système International d'Unités (SI units) for most measurements. This incorporates metric units for mass (*gram*), length (*metre*) and volume (*litre*), which are the most common ones which nurses and midwives have to use. Larger and smaller quantities are given a prefix which denotes whether they are 10, 100, 1000 or 1,000,000 times bigger or smaller than the basic unit. These prefixes can be applied to any of the metric units as seen in Table 3.1, but only the terms which you are likely to use as a nurse or midwife are shown. Strictly speaking, the *kilogram* is the base unit of mass, but for the purposes of explaining relative size of units, here we will consider the gram as the starting point for measurement of mass.

Table 3.1 indicates the relationship between the various measures. *Kilo* is used as a prefix for a value 1000 times the basic unit. One

Table 3.1 Commonly used metric measurements and their relationship to the basic unit

Kilo	Basic Unit	Centi	Milli	Micro	Nano
× 1000 (10^3)	× 1	× 0.01 (10^{-2})	× 0.001 (10^{-3})	× 0.000001 (10^{-6})	× 0.000000001 (10^{-9})
kilogram (kg)	gram (g)		milligram (mg)	microgram (mcg or µg)	nanogram (ng)
kilometre (km)	metre (m)	Centimetre (cm)	millimetre (mm)	Micrometer (micron)	
	litre (L)		millilitre (mL or ml)		

kilometre is 1000 metres. *Centi* is used to show that a measurement is one-hundredth of the basic unit. A metre is made up of 100 centimetres. (You will come across this prefix in other connotations, for example, centigrade, the scale used to measure temperature; **centiles** used in children's growth charts and as a suffix in *percent*. 'Cent' always suggests that the number one hundred is involved). *Milli* is used to denote 1000th of the basic unit. One millimetre is 0·001 or 1000th of a metre. *Micro* is even smaller and means a millionth of the basic unit. The diameter of a red blood cell is measured in microns.

Where very large or very small numbers are involved, the value may be expressed as a power of 10. This is a form of mathematical shorthand and indicates the number of multiplications or, in the case of negative power, divisions by ten required to reach the number. A kilogram could be written 10^3g, indicating that it is 1g multiplied by 10 × 10 × 10 whereas a milligram could be written 10^{-3}g, the negative power indicating that it is *divided* by 10^3. A nanogram (10^{-9}g) is a tiny measure 1,000,000,000th of a gram and is used for a very small number of specific drugs.

Although the safest way to write a unit of measurement is in full, the abbreviations in Table 3.1 are generally acceptable. Note that it is strongly recommended that microgram (mcg or µg) and nanogram (ng) are written *in full* since their abbreviations are too similar to that of milligram (mg) to be safe. Although the full word may be written as a plural, for example, milligrams, note that the abbreviation is not. Ten milligrams is expressed as 10mg. Millilitres are sometimes abbreviated to mL, as in the British National Formulary (BNF), but you will also see it written as ml and this book will use that convention.

Although it is not recognized as good practice, you may come across a prescription which is written for a drug using a different strength from that dispensed. For example, 0·5g may be prescribed for a drug which is dispensed as 500mg. You need to be able to calculate the correct strength before you can give the drug to the patient. We can do this using an equation:

Worked example 3.3 Converting between metric measures – grams to milligrams

0·5g of a drug is prescribed. The label on the bottle states that each tablet is 500mg. NB Always convert the prescription to the strength of the preparation and not the other way round. So, we are changing the prescription (g) to mg.

Method 1: Remember that with an equation, as long as we do the same thing to both sides, the values remain equal.

We know that   1g = 1000mg

So   0·5g = 500mg (both sides divided by 2)

                    = 1 tablet

Method 2: We know that there are 1000mg in a gram and so by multiplying 0·5g by 1000, we will convert it into milligrams.

To multiply by 1000, move the decimal point 3 spaces to the right (one per nought):

0·5g = 500mg

      = 1 tablet

◆ *Check* that this is a sensible answer. Each tablet contains 500mg and giving one tablet would be appropriate.

Worked example 3.4 Converting between metric measures – micrograms to mg

A prescription is for 2000 microgram. The bottle is labelled as 1mg per tablet. So, we need to change the prescribed dose to mg.

Method 1:

1000 microgram = 1mg = 1 tablet

2000 microgram = 2mg (both sides multiplied by 2)

                    = 2 tablets

Method 2: Change the micrograms to milligrams by dividing by 1000 (move the decimal point 3 places to the left):

2000·0 microgram = 2mg

Each tablet is 1mg, so we need 2 tablets.

In medicines management, you will come across a variety of measurements of weight and volume. Occasionally, the term cubic centimetre (cc) may be used instead of millilitre (ml), particularly when referring to size of syringes, and these measures are used interchangeably. In other words, a 10cc syringe is the same thing as a 10ml syringe.

Drugs may also be dispensed in strengths other than the usual metric measures. For example, some hormones, such as insulin and oxytocin, are measured in units of activity and the prescription will be in a number of units (u). Sometimes these are termed international units (iu).

Other metric units, which you may come across but are unlikely to use in any calculations, are:

Moles and *millimols* (mmol) which are applied to the molecular weight of chemicals and seen in laboratory reports.

Joules which constitute a measure of energy referred to in defibrillator use.

Although the metric unit for pressure is the **Pascal** (Pa), the most common measurement of pressure in healthcare is millimetres (mm) of mercury (Hg) which is used when measuring arterial blood pressure (BP) and Central Venous Pressure (CVP), although CVP is occasionally measured in centimetres (cm) of water (H_2O).

 Practice exercise 3.3 Metric conversion (suitable for all)

1 A prescription is written as 0·25g. What is the equivalent number of milligrams?
2 Convert 7500 microgram to mg.
3 How many millilitres in 1·3 litres?
4 Write 0·025 microgram as nanograms.
5 What is 1250mg expressed in grams?

Check your answers in Appendix E.

Conversion between imperial measures and metric units and vice versa

Although the health profession uses metric units to measure weight and length, the traditional announcement of a new baby usually includes a weight in the old imperial measures of pounds and ounces and often a length in inches. Many people in the UK have also been slow to incorporate the metric system when referring to their own height and weight and so healthcare workers need to be able to convert from one to the other. Although conversion charts exist, these may not always be at hand and so knowing how to do the conversion yourself is useful. Converting between metric and Imperial measures involves calculations which use several of the basic mathematical skills covered in Chapter 2, particularly calculating using decimal fractions. To be able to convert, you also need to know how many imperial units there are in a metric unit and vice versa. Here are some accepted equivalents:

1kg = 2·2lbs (there are 16oz in 1 pound and 14 pounds in 1 stone)

1 metre = 39 inches (12 inches in a foot)

1 fluid ounce = 28·4 millilitres

Worked example 3.5 Converting kilograms to pounds and ounces

Newborn weight = 3·45kg. What is that in pounds and ounces?

First, approximate or estimate by rounding up or down:

1kg is approximately 2lb and 3·45 is nearly 3·5 or $3\frac{1}{2}$.

So 3·5kg will be approximately $3\frac{1}{2} \times 2 = 7$lb.

Now do the actual calculation:

1kg = 2·2lb

3·45kg = 2·2 × 3·45lb

To multiply two decimals, go back to p. 22.

The answer you should get is 7·59lb.

But we have not yet got an amount in pounds *and ounces*. There are 16oz in a lb and so again make an approximation:

0·59 is just over half and so our answer should be just over half a pound or 8oz.

Now do the calculation:

0·59 of 16oz = 0·59 × 16

= 9·44oz this is just over 8 and so is a sensible answer.

So our converted weight is 7lb 9·44oz.

As we do not use anything smaller than an ounce when weighing babies using imperial measures, the 0·44 can be rounded down and the nearest equivalent weight to 3·45kg given as 7lb 9oz.

Worked example 3.6 Converting fluid ounces to millilitres

Infant feeding is another area where the units used by lay people such as parents and the measurements used on Infant Formula preparations are in imperial units (fluid ounces) whereas the hospital is likely to use metric units (millilitres), particularly if the child is very sick and is being tube fed. To get a good idea of what an infant's normal intake is, you may need to convert a mother's reported '7ounce bottle' into millilitres (ml).

To convert from fluid ounces to millilitres:

1 fluid ounce = 28·4 millilitres

So 7 fluid ounces = 7 × 28·4ml

Which gives us 198·8ml, or approximately 200ml.

NB: We accept a rounding up of just over a millilitre in this case, whereas this would not be acceptable if we were dealing with much smaller amounts, especially if these included drugs.

Practice exercise 3.4 Conversion of imperial to metric measures and vice versa (i) (particularly suitable for neonatal nursing and midwifery)

Mrs Allan is delivered of a healthy baby boy whose weight and length are recorded on the birth record as 3·16kg and 49cm. The baby's elderly grandmother does not understand decimals and wants to know what that means in measurements which she can understand, meaning pounds and ounces and inches. You cannot find the conversion chart and so need to calculate these for her.

1 What is 3·16kg in pounds and ounces?

2 What is 49cm in inches? (Correct to the nearest inch)

The baby is weighed again after 2 days and is found to be 3kg exactly. Giving answers correct to 1 decimal place;

3 How much weight has he lost in metric measures?

4 What is the equivalent weight loss in ounces?

At age 5 days, the baby has put on weight and is now 3·25kg.

5 How much weight in ounces has he gained since birth?

Check your answers in Appendix E.

Practice exercise 3.5 Conversion of imperial to metric measures and vice versa (ii) (particularly suitable for Children's and Learning Disability nurses)

James is a 10-year-old boy presenting at the children's hospital for investigations into small stature. He is weighed and measured with the following results: Weight = 26·5kg, Height = 115cm. Giving answers to nearest pound or nearest inch;

1 What is James's weight in stones and pounds?

2 How tall is James in feet and inches?

James's twin brother Michael is weighed and measured at the same visit. His results are: Weight = 40kg, Height = 145cm

3 Convert Michael's weight to imperial measures.

4 How much taller is he than James (in inches)?

Check your answers in Appendix E.

Practice exercise 3.6 Conversion of imperial to metric measures and vice versa (iii) (suitable for all)

Hamish Jameson, aged 17, has a chromosomal abnormality, is 5 foot 2 inches tall and tells you that he weighs 11 stone 12lbs. The unit's weighing scales are out of order and the conversion charts are missing and so you need to convert his weight into kilograms and height into centimetres for an initial entry to his notes.

1 What is the metric equivalent of 11 stone 12 lbs? (Correct to 1 decimal place)

2 What is 5 foot 5 inches in centimetres?

Hamish is put on a low carbohydrate diet and 4 weeks later is reweighed on the new scales which register 72kg. Giving answers to the nearest lb:

3 How much weight has he lost?

4 What is Hamish's new weight in imperial measures?

Check your answers in Appendix E.

Graphs

There are many types of graph, but most used in everyday health-care practice are modified line graphs. These are used in nursing and midwifery practice to plot changes in a patient's condition, as on a patient's observation chart, or to compare measurements with normal values as in a children's growth chart.

Line graphs are arranged on two intersecting axes with independent scales, for example, temperature can be plotted against time or changes in weight against calorific intake. The observation chart shows changes in the patient's condition over time and can be helpful in identifying not only the presence of fever (a high temperature) but the nature of the possible underlying infection. For example, some infections cause a higher temperature in the evening. The observation chart can also indicate the effectiveness of medication given to reduce blood pressure, bring down the temperature or steady a rapid pulse rate.

Hence, understanding what the lines on the graph mean and accurate plotting of a measurement on the chart are important. Figures 3.1 to 3.3 show children's growth charts for different sexes and ages and a symphysis-fundal height chart, used in midwifery. These charts are also called centile charts for reasons which will become apparent.

This type of graph is useful for plotting changing parameters such as a child's weight or height over time. A children's growth chart can be consulted to gauge whether a child is growing too slowly or quickly in comparison with accepted norms. If a measure, such as height, is on the 5th centile, this means that for every 100 children of that age, 5 (5%) would be expected to be shorter and 95 (95%) would be expected to be taller. This is not indicative of normality or otherwise from a single reading, but plotting a particular child's height and/or weight over time can be a useful indication of health. In midwifery practice the symphysis-fundal height chart may be used to help plot the growth of the foetus.

Worked example 3.7 Using growth charts

To assess a female baby of 3 months whose weight is 6kg, we look at the relevant chart shown in Figure 3.1 to see where the 3-month line intersects with the 6kg line. This is exactly on the 75th centile as marked on this chart, which means that for every 100 female children at 3 months of age, 25 are likely to weigh more than 6kg and 74 will weigh less than 6kg.

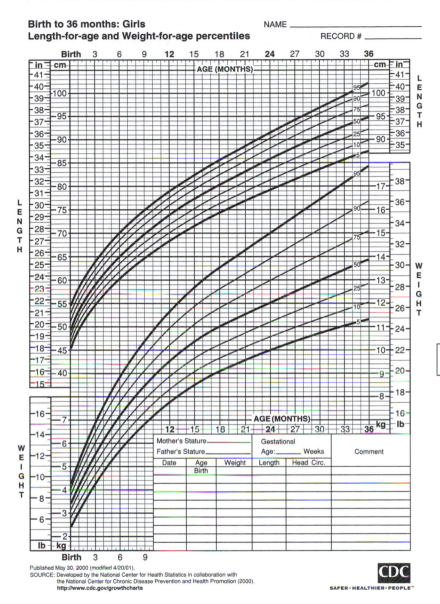

Birth to 36 months: Girls
Length-for-age and Weight-for-age percentiles

NAME _____

RECORD # _____

Published May 30, 2000 (modified 4/20/01).
SOURCE: Developed by the National Center for Health Statistics in collaboration with
the National Center for Chronic Disease Prevention and Health Promotion (2000).
http://www.cdc.gov/growthcharts

CDC
SAFER · HEALTHIER · PEOPLE™

Figure 3.1 Growth chart for girls, 0–36 months

If we assess the same child at 12 months, we could expect her weight to be on the same centile which would mean that at 12 months she should weigh about 10·2kg.

Practice exercise 3.7 Growth charts (i) (suitable for all but particularly midwives, children's nurses and health visitors)

Use the Girls birth to 36 months growth chart (Figure 3.1) to answer the following:

1 On what centile for weight is a girl who is born at term weighing 4kg?

2 At 12 months she weighs 9·5kg. Which centile does this represent?

3 A healthy 9-month-old baby girl is 65cm. Approximately what height would you expect her to reach by the age of 2 years?

Check your answers in Appendix E.

Practice exercise 3.8 Symphysis-fundal height chart (midwifery)

Use the symphysis-fundal height chart (Figure 3.2) to answer the following:

Mrs Jones is 19 weeks pregnant and has her fundal height plotted on the symphysis-fundal height chart. It is 20cm.

1 Which centile does this measurement lie on?

2 If she continues on this centile, what height will her fundus be expected to reach at 36 weeks?

3 What does this centile measurement indicate?

Check your answers in Appendix E.

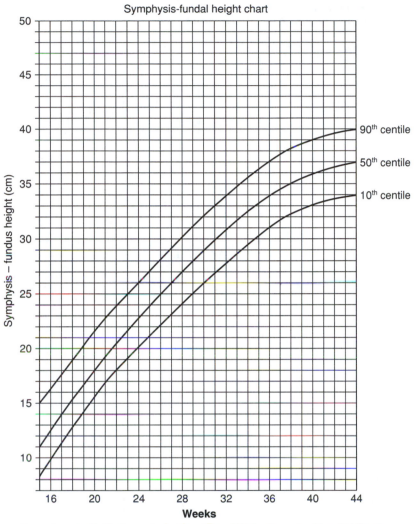

Symphysis-fundal height chart

Reproduced with kind permission from Royal Wolverhampton Hospital Trust

Figure 3.2 Symphysis-fundal height chart

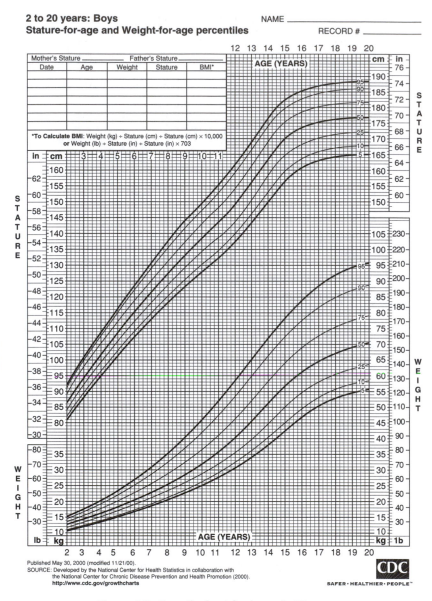

2 to 20 years: Boys
Stature-for-age and Weight-for-age percentiles

NAME _____

RECORD # _____

50

Published May 30, 2000 (modified 11/21/00).
SOURCE: Developed by the National Center for Health Statistics in collaboration with
the National Center for Chronic Disease Prevention and Health Promotion (2000).
http://www.cdc.gov/growthcharts

CDC
SAFER · HEALTHIER · PEOPLE™

Figure 3.3 Growth chart for boys, 2–20 years

Practice exercise 3.9 Growth charts (ii) (suitable for all but particularly children's nurses)

Use the Boys 2–20 years growth chart (Figure 3.3) to answer the following:

Timmy is an 8-year-old boy. His weight = 20kg and height = 118cm. Compare Timmy's measurements with the growth chart for Boys 2–20 years.

1 On which centile does Timmy's height measurement lie?

2 Is his weight on the same centile as his height?

3 What would you tell his parents about these findings?

Check your answers in Appendix E.

Practice exercise 3.10 Growth charts (iii) (suitable for Adult, Learning Disability and Mental Health nurses)

Use the Boys 2–20 years growth chart (Figure 3.3) to answer the following:

John is 17 years old. He is 163cm tall and weighs 89kg.

1 What centile is John on for height?

2 Which centile is he on for weight?

3 What does this indicate?

Check your answers in Appendix E.

The measurements explored in this chapter are typical of those used in healthcare practice. The following chapters cover medication and fluid prescriptions which use some of these measurements in different ways.

4 Medications Safety: Tablets and Capsules

This chapter covers:

◆ The prescription

◆ The importance of estimation

◆ Different ways to calculate medication dosage

◆ Formulae – how to construct and use them

◆ Checking your calculation

One of the most common calculations that a nurse or midwife has to do is working out the correct medication to give from a prescription. There are several elements to this skill, only one of which is the actual calculation, but all of which are important. You have already learnt how to convert prescriptions from one strength to another and have done some basic calculations. However, this book has been written chiefly to help you with the calculation side of medicines management and this is what this chapter will cover.

When preparing to work out a medication dose, the first thing is to make sure that you understand the prescription and extract the information essential for your calculation.

Let's look at the fundamental information on any prescription, be it on a prescriber's pad (Figure 4.1) or a purpose-made hospital prescription sheet (Figure 4.2).

The information on the prescription that concerns us in relation to calculating drug dosage is:

◆ the name of the drug;

◆ the format of the drug and route of administration;

◆ the strength of the drug;

◆ the time period over which it is to be given. Note that the way this is written will vary from place to place. Although explicit directions in English are recommended, some prescribers still use Latin abbreviations. These can be found in Appendix A.

Pharmacy stamp	Age: 1 year 11 months Date of birth 4/6/2006	Title, forename, surname & address Miss Lucy Patient 12 Anyold Street Hopetown HO4 5PE
Number of days' treatment NB Ensure dose is stated	5	

Endorsements	Amoxicillin oral suspension 125mg/5ml sugar-free 125mg three times daily Supply 100ml (No more items on this prescription)

Signature of prescriber Michael Dogood	Date 02/05/08

For dispenser No. of Prescriptions on form	Anyborough Health Authority Dr. M. Dogood 123 High Street Hopetown HO1 2PZ Tel: 0111 222 233

NHS

XXXXXXXX

Figure 4.1 Example of a prescription on NHS prescriber's pad

53

Hosp no. xxxxxxx	D.O.B. 11/02/1978	SAINT SUNDAY HOSPITAL	**NHS**
Surname	Patient		
First names	Kevin John	Ward: 12	
Address	12, Anyold Street,	Consultant: Mr. Surgeon	
	Hopetown,	Chart number: 1	
	HO4 5PE	Number of Charts in use: 1	

PRESCRIPTION CHART

ALLERGIES and DRUG SENSITIVITIES		Patient's own drugs:
Elastoplast		

Height 195cm	Weight 71kg	Date of admission: 05/06/2008

ONCE ONLY AND PRE-MEDICATION DRUGS

Date	Name of drug	Dose	Route	Time to be given	Signature	Given by	Time given	Pharm
06/06/08	TEMAZEPAM	20mg	Oral	07.00	GAMann			

AS REQUIRED AND POST OPERATIVE DRUGS

DRUG APPROVED NAME TRAMADOL	Dose 50mg	Route O	Dose	Date	Time	Dose	Given	Dose	Date	Time	Dose	Given
			1					8				
Frequency QDS	Indication PAIN	Date 6/06/08	Pharm	2				9				
				3				10				
Number of doses	Detailed directions			4				11				
6				5				12				
Prescriber's signature	Review pain chart			6				13				
GAMann				7				14				

REGULAR DRUGS

			Date →								
			Time	Dose							
DRUG APPROVED NAME	Route	Frequency									
PHENYTOIN	Oral	Daily	0700								
Prescriber's signature	Bleep	Pharm	1000								
GAMann	2664		1200								
Detailed directions	Date written 06/06/08		1400								
Nocté			1700								
	Date cancelled		2200	300mg							

DRUG APPROVED NAME	Route	Frequency									
AMOXICILLIN	Oral	QDS	0700	500mg							
Prescriber's signature	Bleep	Pharm	1000								
GAMann	2664		1200	500mg							
Detailed directions	Date written 06/06/08		1400								
			1700	500mg							
	Date cancelled		2200	500mg							

Figure 4.2 Pages from a typical hospital drug chart

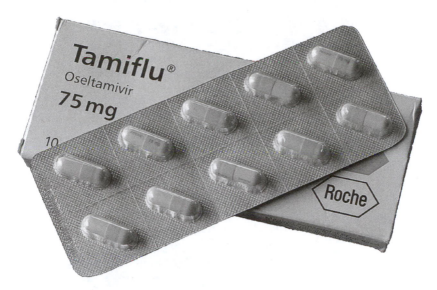

Figure 4.3 Illustration of drug packaging

Second, you need to look at the *label* on the medicine container and extract the information that you need in order to work out what you have to give. Information on the label will include:

◆ the name of the drug;

◆ the dose per tablet/capsule/caplet;

◆ the number of items in the pack (pre-packed medicines only).

NB: Each drug has an approved name (which is universal) but many also have a manufacturer's name which is specific to them. Drugs supplied as 'generics' only have an approved name. An example of this is Diclofenac Sodium slow release capsules which are manufactured as Diclomax SR by Provalis and as Rheumalgan SR by Sandoz. Although packaged differently, both have the same active ingredients.

In Figure 4.3, Tamiflu is the proprietary or manufacturer's name, but Oseltamivir is the approved name.

Some labels or *names* of substances may include numbers or percentages as part of the labelling and this can be confusing, for example, 0·9% normal saline or 5% dextrose. So make sure you understand what numbers relate to the name of the substance and which are relevant in deciding the strength or dosage. Labels should

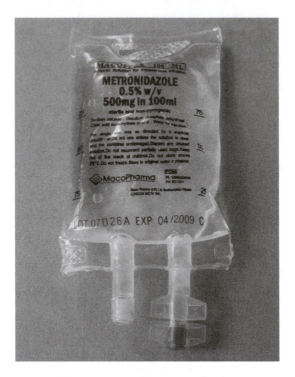

Figure 4.4 Numbers on packaging

also include an expiry date for the contents (see Figure 4.4). Although the expiry date is usually in numbers, and is important in that you do not give out-of-date medicines, these numbers are not relevant to any calculation of dosage.

Common sense and estimation

The golden rule of any calculation you make is to have a good idea of what a sensible answer should be. This is much easier with experience, but you will soon develop 'common-sense' knowledge if you are reflective in your own practice. As well as 'common-sense knowing', you need to make a habit of estimating, especially if the calculation involves decimals or several stages, or if you are using a hand-held calculator (see Chapter 1). Another estimate should be based on the recommended dose range in the formulary in use locally, especially if you are in a new workplace or faced with an unfamiliar substance.

In the case of medication calculations, you are just as accountable as the prescriber and it is not safe to assume that the prescription is automatically correct. Administering an erroneous prescription is committing a medication error just as much as writing an erroneous prescription.

Ways of calculating medication dosage

Many calculations required in nursing and midwifery are so straight-forward that mental arithmetic is all that you need. There are several ways of calculating medication dosages using mental arithmetic and you may feel more comfortable using one than another.

Unit dose

The most straightforward calculations are at unit dose level. In other words, the prescribed dose is the same as the dispensed medicine. Look at this example of a prescription for an antibiotic:

Date	Name of drug	Dose	Route	Frequency
10/02/08	TETRACYCLINE	250mg	oral	6 hrly

The label on the bottle is

> Tetracycline Tabs
> 250mg

Having checked that the prescription is in the same units (mg) as the dispensed drug, we can see immediately that we need one tablet to give the prescribed dose of 250mg. So, we don't really need to do a calculation. This is termed a unit dose.

Calculations are really only needed when the prescription is at sub- or multiple unit level. In other words, when the prescribed amount is less than the dispensed preparation, or more than the dispensed unit. Let's look at what that really means.

Multiple unit dose

Date	Name of drug	Dose	Route	Frequency
10/02/08	TETRACYCLINE	500mg	oral	q.d.s.

The label on the bottle is:

> Tetracycline Tabs
> 250mg

In this case, the prescribed dose is twice the amount which is contained in one tablet. Common sense tells us that we will need to give 2 tablets, but what if the calculation is not so straightforward? Let's look at an example.

Worked example 4.1 Multiple unit dose

A patient is prescribed an oral drug for control of diabetes.

Date	Name of drug	Dose	Route	Frequency
10/02/08	CHLORPROPAMIDE	250mg	oral	daily

This would normally be given as a unit dose using one 250mg strength tablet. In this scenario, the only tablets available are these. How many tablets do we need to give?

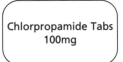

> Chlorpropamide Tabs
> 100mg

◆ *Extract* the required information from the prescription and the label:

We need to give 250mg and what we have is tablets, each containing 100mg.

◆ *Check*: Is the stock medicine in the same units as the prescribed dose?

Yes, both stock and prescription are in milligrams.

◆ *Estimate*: Do you need more or less than the stock dosage?

As 250 is larger than 100, we will need more than 1 tablet (100mg) and indeed more than 2 (200mg), but less than 3 (300mg).

◆ *Calculate the dose:*

Method 1: Look for relationships between the numbers involved. You may see immediately that 250 is $2\frac{1}{2}$ times 100 and that you will need to give $2\frac{1}{2}$ tablets.

Or

Method 2: You could reason that if one tablet contains 100mg, then 2 tablets will contain 200mg and $\frac{1}{2}$ a tablet will contain 50mg. Thus, $2\frac{1}{2}$ tablets will provide the required amount of 250mg.

Or if you need another way of calculating the dose.

Method 3: If you know what contains 1mg of the drug, then you can multiply it by 250 to find what you need to give for the pre-scribed dose. So, if 100mg is contained in 1 tablet, make this into an equation:

100mg = 1 tablet

Divide both sides of the equation by 100

$$1\text{mg} = \frac{1}{100} \text{ of a tablet}$$

Then multiply both sides by 250:

$$250\text{mg} = \frac{1}{100} \times \frac{250}{1}$$

$$= \frac{25}{10}$$

$$= 2\cdot5 \text{ tablets } (2\tfrac{1}{2})$$

Method 3 may seem a complicated method for this straightforward calculation, but it gives you a way of tackling those which are more difficult.

Whichever method you use, *check* that your answer is around the estimated amount and is a sensible amount to be given by the pre-scribed route. In this case, we estimated that we needed more than 2 tablets and less than 3, and so our answer of $2\frac{1}{2}$ tablets is reasonable.

NB: Breaking tablets in half is not considered good practice and should only be done if the tablets are scored and no alternative strength is available. Under no circumstances should you attempt to break enteric coated (e/c) tablets.

Practice exercise 4.1 Multiple unit drug calculations (i) (suitable for all)

Using any of the above methods, work out the number of tablets/capsules required for the following prescriptions, using the stock as per labels supplied:

1 John has bipolar disorder. This is an excerpt from his prescription.

Name of drug	Dose	Route
VALPROIC ACID (DEPAKOTE)	500mg	oral

2 Mrs Hall suffers from rheumatic disease and is prescribed this non-steroidal anti-inflammatory drug.

Name of drug	Dose	Route
NAPROXEN	0·5g	oral

3 Mr Conlon has a severe Vitamin B₁ deficiency. This is taken from his prescription.

Name of drug	Dose	Route
THIAMINE	150mg	oral

4 Julie has been prescribed this steroid to relieve her angio-oedema.

Name of drug	Dose	Route
DEXAMETHASONE	1mg	oral

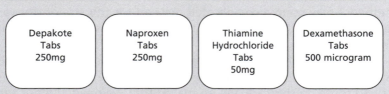

Depakote Tabs 250mg | Naproxen Tabs 250mg | Thiamine Hydrochloride Tabs 50mg | Dexamethasone Tabs 500 microgram

NB: You may have noticed that the prescription for Thiamine is just 'Thiamine' while the tablets are labelled 'Thiamine hydrochloride'. The additional part of the label indicates how the active drug is prepared and should not alter the active ingredient. If in doubt, check with the prescriber or refer to a reputable formulary for confirmation that you have the correct preparation.

Check your answers in Appendix E.

Sub-unit dose

The dose for a child or elderly person is often less than the unit dose. We can use the same methods to calculate sub-unit dose as we did for multiple unit doses.

Worked example 4.2 Sub-unit dose

Take the prescription below for an oral preparation of an anti-emetic.

Date	Name of drug	Dose	Route	Frequency
10/02/08	CYCLIZINE	25mg	oral	8 hrly

The label on the bottle of tablets is:

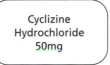

Cyclizine
Hydrochloride
50mg

- *Extract* the required information from the prescription and the label:

  We need to give 25mg and what we have is tablets, each of 50mg.

- *Check*: Is the stock medicine in the same units as the prescribed dose?

  Yes, both stock and prescription are in mg.

- *Estimate*: Do you need more or less than the stock dosage?

  As 25 is smaller than 50, we will need less than 1 tablet.

- *Calculate the dose*:

  Method 1: Look for relationships between the numbers involved. You can probably see immediately that 25 is $\frac{1}{2}$ of 50 and that you will need to give $\frac{1}{2}$ a tablet.

  Or

  Method 2: You could reason that if one tablet contains 50mg, then $\frac{1}{2}$ tablet will contain 25mg (this is what you are unconsciously doing in method 1).

  Or

  Method 3: If you know what contains 1mg of the drug, then you can multiply it by 25 to find what you need to give for the prescribed dose.

So, if 50mg is contained in 1 tablet:

1mg will be in $\dfrac{1}{50}$ of a tablet

And 25mg in $\dfrac{25}{1} \times \dfrac{1}{50} = \dfrac{25}{50} = \dfrac{1}{2}$ tablet

Whatever method used, the prescription is for 25mg, which is half the unit dose of 50mg per tablet and so we need to give half a tablet.

Practice exercise 4.2 Sub-unit drug calculations (suitable for all)

Again using any of the above methods, work out the required dose for the following prescriptions using the stock as per labels supplied:

1 To prevent episodes of self-harm, Peter is prescribed a daily dose of an anti-manic drug:

Name of drug	Dose	Route
LITHIUM	125mg	oral

2 Frances has been prescribed this steroid to relieve urticaria:

Name of drug	Dose	Route
HYDROCORTISONE	15mg	oral

3 Mrs Little needs help with bladder control. She is prescribed:

Name of drug	Dose	Route
OXYBUTYNIN HYDROCHLORIDE (CYSTRIN)	2·5mg	oral

Lithium Carbonate Tabs 250mg	Hydrocortisone Tabs 10mg	Cystrin Tabs 5mg

Check your answers in Appendix E.

NB: Remember that although these tablets are scored and therefore suitable for breaking into two, it is not considered good practice to give broken tablets. Avoid doing this if possible, these examples are given for calculation practice (there is often a liquid preparation available which will give more reliable measures of the drug). Never attempt to break tablets that are not scored.

Using a formula

As you can see, medication dosage calculations take the form of an equation where one side equals the other. As you have seen, there is no single right way to calculate drug dosages, but there *is* one *formula*, in the form of an equation that always works.

The worked examples below of easy calculations will show you how the formula is made up and if you forget how to set it up, you can always work it out using a calculation which is very easy, such as these.

Worked example 4.3 Multiple unit dose

The patient is prescribed Levothyroxine (Thyroxine) for hypothyroidism.

Date	Name of drug	Dose	Route	Frequency
10/02/08	LEVOTHYROXINE	50 micrograms	oral	once daily

This is supplied in tablet form:

Label on bottle:

> Levothyroxine
> Tabs
> 25 micrograms

◆ *Extract* the required information from the prescription and the label:

We need to give 50 microgram and have got 25 microgram tablets.

◆ *Check*: Is the stock medicine in the same units as the prescribed dose?

Yes, stock and prescription are in the same units (micrograms).

◆ *Estimate*: Do we need more or less than the stock dosage?

The prescription is for 50 microgram and the unit dose is 25 microgram so we will need more than one tablet.

♦ *Calculate*

Method 1: The prescribed dose of 50 microgram is twice the stock strength of 25 microgram per tablet and this means the patient should be given 2 tablets.

Method 2: If 1 tablet contains 25 microgram, then 2 tablets will contain twice as much, in other words, 50 micrograms which is the prescribed dose.

Let's look closer at how you got the answer in each of these methods:

The *dose prescribed*, or *what you want*, was 50 micrograms.

The *stock dose* available, or *what you have*, was 25 micrograms.

To reach the correct answer of 2 tablets, you divided 50 by 25.

The third method that we have used shows this even more clearly.

Method 3: If 25mg = 1 tablet

$$1mg = \frac{1}{25} \text{ tablet}$$

$$50mg = \frac{1}{25} \times \frac{50}{1} = \frac{50}{25}$$

The numerator and denominator are numbers that you will almost certainly recognize as being related. Both are divisible by 25 and 5. If you couldn't see immediately that 50 divided by 25 was 2, then you could break the fraction down by dividing both top and bottom by 5 to get $\frac{10}{5}$:

So, 50mg = 2 tablets

♦ *Check* that your answer is around the estimated amount and is a sensible amount to be given by the prescribed route.

Worked example 4.4 Sub-unit dose

To prevent travel sickness, a 9-year-old child is prescribed Promethazine Teoclate.

Date	Name of drug	Dose	Route	Time to be given
10/02/08	PROMETHAZINE TEOCLATE	12·5mg	oral	1 hour before travel

MEDICATIONS SAFETY: TABLETS AND CAPSULES

Label on the bottle of scored tablets:

> Promethazine
> Teoclate
> Tabs 25mg

- *Extract* the required information from the prescription and the label:
  Prescription is for 12·5mg and we have stock of 25mg tablets.
- *Check*: Is the stock medicine in the same units as the prescribed dose?
  Yes, stock and prescription are the same units (milligrams).
- *Estimate*: Do you need more or less than the stock dosage?
  The prescription is for 12·5mg and the unit dose is 25mg and so we will need less than one tablet.
- *Calculate*

  Method 1: The stock strength of 25mg per tablet is twice the prescribed dose of 12·5mg and this means that the patient should be given half a tablet.

  Method 2: If 1 tablet contains 25mg, then half a tablet will contain half as much, in other words, 12·5mg.

Again, let's look closer at how you got the answer in each of these methods:

The *dose prescribed*, or *what you want*, was 12·5mg.

The *dose per available tablet*, or *what you have*, was 25mg.

To reach the correct answer of $\frac{1}{2}$ tablet, you divided 12·5 by 25.

Method 3:

If 25mg = 1 tablet

$$1\text{mg} = \frac{1}{25} \text{ tablet}$$

$$12\cdot5\text{mg} = \frac{1}{25} \times 12\cdot5 \text{ or } \frac{12\cdot5}{25}$$

The resulting fraction can be simplified by cancelling down and dividing both top and bottom by 25 or if you prefer, by 5 (twice):

$$\frac{\overset{2\cdot5}{\cancel{12\cdot5}}}{\underset{5}{\cancel{25}}} = \frac{\overset{0\cdot5}{\cancel{2\cdot5}}}{\underset{1}{\cancel{5}}} = 0\cdot5$$

0·5 is, of course $\frac{1}{2}$ tablet.

Alternatively, we could get rid of the decimal in $\frac{12.5}{25}$ by multiplying top and bottom by 10:

So $12 \cdot 5\text{mg} = \dfrac{125}{250}$

Again, cancelling down by 5s or 25 will eventually give us $\frac{1}{2}$ tablet.

◆ *Check* that your answer is around the estimated amount and is a sensible amount to be given by the prescribed route.

Hence, for both sub-unit and multi-unit dosages, we could add to our calculating methods and substitute known values into the formula below, remembering that you must have the same units top and bottom:

$$\dfrac{\textit{What you want}}{\textit{What you've got}} = \text{dose (in tablets)}$$

You should carry out all basic medication dosage calculations following these stages:

◆ *Extract* the relevant information from the prescription.

◆ *Check* that the drug is available in the same units as the prescription.

◆ *Estimate* an approximate answer.

◆ *Calculate using your chosen method* (see above).

◆ *Check this answer* against the approximation from step 3 and check that it is a sensible format and amount to be given by the route prescribed.

You will notice that many of the dosage calculations involve similar numbers. This is because medications are usually both prescribed and prepared in round numbers which are easy to calculate. Part of the 'common-sense' element to drug calculation is recognizing these numbers and the relationships between them.

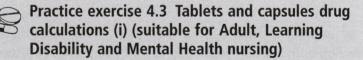

Practice exercise 4.3 Tablets and capsules drug calculations (i) (suitable for Adult, Learning Disability and Mental Health nursing)

Use any of the methods discussed in this chapter to calculate the required medication doses as given below. The labels on the medicine bottles are shown below each prescription.

On Friday you are working on a ward with elderly patients and have been asked to help the registered nurse by giving out the morning medicines to the patients in the four-bedded unit to which you are allocated. Your mentor asks you to calculate each dose yourself before checking with her.

					MARY SMITH: D.O.B. 25/02/21
	Date	Name of drug	Dose	Route	Frequency
1	10/02/08	Cefalexin	500mg	oral	twice daily (b.d.)
2	10/02/08	Tolbutamide	0·5g	oral	once a day (8am)

Cefalexin Caps
250mg

Tolbutamide
Tabs
500mg

					JANE FIELD: D.O.B. 14/04/34
	Date	Name of drug	Dose	Route	Frequency
3	06/02/08	Methotrexate	7·5mg	oral	Every Friday 8am
4	06/02/08	Diclofenac Sodium	50mg	oral	b.d.

Methotrexate
Tabs
2·5mg

Diclofenac Sodium
Tabs
25mg

					RITA SISSONS: D.O.B. 21/12/25
	Date	Name of drug	Dose	Route	Frequency
5	06/02/08	Tramadol Hydrochloride	100mg	oral	4 hrly p.r.n.
6	06/02/08	Cyclizine Hydrochloride	25mg	oral	t.d.s.

Tramadol
Hydrochloride
Caps
50mg

Cyclizine
Hydrochloride
Tabs (scored)
50mg

Check your answers in Appendix E.

Practice exercise 4.4 Tablets and capsules drug calculations (ii) (suitable for midwifery)

Calculate the doses required by the following patients:

Joanne Lum's previous pregnancy resulted in a stillborn child with a neural tube defect. She is in very early pregnancy and has been admitted for bed rest as her blood pressure is high.

					JOANNE LUM: D.O.B. 24/02/77
	Date	**Name of drug**	**Dose**	**Route**	**Frequency**
1	06/02/08	FOLIC ACID	4mg	oral	once a day
2	06/02/08	METHYLDOPA	250mg	oral	b.d.

Folic Acid
Tabs
400 microgram

Methyldopa
Tabs
125mg

Mrs Divi is post-partum but has an infection and needs antibiotics and pain control.

					LEILA DIVI: D.O.B. 03/09/86
	Date	**Name of drug**	**Dose**	**Route**	**Frequency**
3	06/02/08	CEFADROXIL	0·5g	oral	b.d.
4	06/02/08	PARACETAMOL	1g	oral	6 hrly p.r.n.

Cefadroxil
Caps
500mg

Paracetamol
Tabs
500mg

Check your answers in Appendix E.

This chapter has dealt with tablets and capsules, but not all medication is in solid format. In the next chapter we will look at calculations related to liquid medicines and doses based on body weight.

5 Medications Safety: Liquid Medication and Prescriptions Based on Weight

This chapter covers:

◆ Liquid medications

◆ Additional checks for children and the elderly

◆ Taking weight into consideration

Liquid medications

We have already looked at different ways of how to calculate straight-forward prescriptions for tablets and capsules. You may have noticed that very few children's examples were given. This is because many drugs used on children are prepared as liquids. This makes them easier to give in a range of doses, as would be required by children of different ages and sizes. The same methods that we used for calculating tablets and capsules can be applied to calculate liquid medicines. But how does the formula which we devised in the previous chapter work for liquids? Let's look at an example.

Worked example 5.1 Liquid medication (i)

A toddler is prescribed the antibiotic Flucloxacillin for an ear infection.

Date	Name of drug	Dose	Route	Frequency
10/02/08	FLUCLOXACILLIN	125mg	oral	4 × daily

Label on bottle:

> Flucloxacillin Syrup
> 125mg in 5ml

This drug is available in syrup form, 125mg in 5ml. This is the unit dose, the liquid equivalent of 1 tablet. How much should you give?

◆ *Extract* the relevant information from the prescription.

◆ *Check* that the drug is available in the same units as the prescription.

◆ *Estimate* an approximate answer.

The answer is of course 5ml.
    But what if the prescription is for a different amount?

Date	Name of drug	Dose	Route	Frequency
10/02/08	FLUCLOXACILLIN	250mg	oral	4 × daily

This drug is available in syrup form, 125mg in 5ml. How much should you give?

◆ *Extract* the relevant information from the prescription.

◆ *Check* that the drug is available in the same units as the prescription.

◆ *Estimate* an approximate answer. The prescribed dose of 250mg is more than the unit dose on the bottle and so we will need more than 5ml.

◆ *Calculate* using your chosen method:

Method 1: You can probably see that 250 is twice 125 and so a dose of 10ml (twice the 'unit' 5ml) is required.

Method 2: If 5ml contains 125mg, then we need twice as much (10ml) to get 250mg.

Method 3: If 125mg = 5ml

$$1mg = \frac{5}{125}ml$$

$$250mg = \frac{5}{125} \times 250ml$$

$$250mg = \frac{1250}{125}ml$$

$$250mg = 10ml$$

Would using the formula (*Method 4*) give this answer?

Method 4: Apply the formula: $\dfrac{\textit{what you want}}{\textit{what you've got}} = \text{dose}$

Substitute the known values to get your answer:

$$\frac{what\ you\ want}{what\ you've\ got} = \frac{250}{125}$$

Dividing top and bottom by 25 $\dfrac{\cancel{250}^{10}}{\cancel{125}_{5}}$

or by 5 several times if you prefer $\dfrac{\cancel{250}^{\cancel{50}^{10}}}{\cancel{125}_{\cancel{25}_{5}}}$ gives $\dfrac{10}{5} = 2$

And so the answer is 2.

♦ *Check this answer* against the approximation from step 3 and check that it is a sensible format and amount to be given by the route prescribed. We estimated that the dose would be more than 5ml and so 2*ml* cannot be right. So our answer is two 'whats'.

Remember that each 125mg dose of what we have *is contained in 5ml* and so the answer is two lots of 5ml, in other words, 10ml. So, to get a sensible answer, we have to multiply by the measure that the available drug is in. In the previous chapter we were dealing with tablets and capsules where the unit dose was always *one* tablet or capsule and so we were effectively multiplying by 1. Let's add this to the formula to make it work for every type of prescription:

$$\text{Dose} = \frac{what\ you\ want}{what\ you've\ got} \times \frac{what\ it's\ in}{1}$$

Remember that we can put a 1 in the denominator to make it look more like a balanced equation, because any number divided by 1 does not itself change, i.e. $4 \div 1 = 4$.

Check by substituting the values we have above:

$$\text{Dose} = \frac{250}{125} \times \frac{5}{1}$$

Cancel down to simplify, for example, we can divide top and bottom by 25 to get $\frac{10}{5} \times \frac{5}{1}$.

We can simplify further, by cancelling the 5s top and bottom to leave $\frac{10}{1} = 10$. So, the dose required is 10ml.

♦ *Check*: Is this a sensible answer close to our estimate? Yes.

Let's try using the revised formula again, this time for a sub-unit dose.

Worked example 5.2 Liquid medication (ii)

Date	Name of drug	Dose	Route	Frequency
10/02/08	PARACETAMOL	100mg	oral	4 × daily

Label on bottle is:

> Paracetamol
> Oral Suspension
> 120mg in 5ml

- *Extract* the relevant information from the prescription.
- *Check* that the drug is available in the same units as the prescription.
- *Estimate* an approximate answer:

  The prescribed dose of 100mg is less than the unit dose on the bottle and so we will need less than 5ml.

- *Calculate* by applying the revised formula:

$$\text{Dose} = \frac{what\ you\ want}{what\ you've\ got} \times \frac{what\ it's\ in}{1}$$

Substitute the known quantities:

$$\text{Dose} = \frac{100}{120} \times \frac{5}{1}\text{ml}$$

Cancel down by dividing top and bottom by 10 to get:

$$\frac{10}{12} \times \frac{5}{1}\text{ml}$$

Then multiply across both the top line and the bottom line:

$$= \frac{50}{12}\text{ml}$$

$$= 4\frac{2}{12}\text{ml}$$

Two twelfths or one sixth of a millilitre is too small to measure accurately, so the safest thing to do is to round it down to 4ml.

- *Check*: Is this a sensible answer close to our estimate? Yes.

NB: When preparing liquid medicines, especially for children, the amounts may be quite small and in these cases it is recommended that you measure them using a suitable syringe, rather than the conventional medicine pot.

Practice exercise 5.1 Oral liquid medication (suitable for all)

Look at the excerpts from prescriptions below and calculate the dosage according to the labels shown for the dispensed preparations:

1 Martin James is suffering from psychosis and requires night sedation. He refuses to swallow tablets and so is prescribed liquid Chlorpromazine.

Name of drug	Dose	Route
CHLORPROMAZINE HYDROCHLORIDE	75mg	oral

2 An elderly Asian gentleman, Abdul Rhamid has been diagnosed with tuberculosis. This is one of the regime of drugs he is prescribed.

Name of drug	Dose	Route
RIFAMPICIN	150mg	oral

3 Jane Vane has severe vomiting in pregnancy and has been prescribed an anti-emetic.

Name of drug	Dose	Route
METOCHLOPRAMIDE HYDROCHLORIDE	7·5mg	oral

4 Cameron is a child undergoing treatment for cancer in which vomiting is a side-effect. He is prescribed the same anti-emetic.

Name of drug	Dose	Route
METOCHLOPRAMIDE HYDROCHLORIDE	2mg	oral

73

Chlorpromazine Hydrochloride Oral Solution 25mg in 5ml

Rifampicin Syrup 100mg in 5ml

Metochlopramide Hydrochloride Oral Solution 5mg in 5ml

Check your answers in Appendix E.

Additional check before dispensing medications to children or the elderly

Normal adult doses of medications are obviously unsuitable in the majority of cases for children. They may also be unsuitable for very small, frail, or elderly adults. There is an additional check we can do against the prescription which is useful in adult nursing and strongly recommended in children's nursing or if nursing the elderly. This check is an absolute must for prescribers but also safeguards the person giving the medication from dosage errors made in the prescription:

Use the recommended dose range and/or recommended maximum dose given in the local formulary to check that the prescribed amount is sensible, remembering to take into account the size of the patient, route prescribed and frequency of the dose.

Worked example 5.3 Additional check for the elderly

Look at the extract from the prescription chart of an elderly patient newly diagnosed with Alzheimer's disease.

Date	Name of drug	Dose	Route	Frequency
10/02/08	RIVASTIGMINE	1·5mg	oral (by syringe)	twice daily (b.d.)

◆ *Extract* the relevant information from the prescription:

Drug name Rivastigmine (used to treat mild dementia in Alzheimer's disease)

Liquid format to be given orally

Dose 1·5mg

◆ *Check the prescription* especially if unfamiliar with the drug or dealing with children or the elderly:

The British National Formulary (BNF) suggests an initial dose of 1·5mg Rivastigmine twice daily, increasing to usual range of 3–6mg twice daily and maximum 6mg twice daily.

Does this prescription fall within the recommended range?

Yes, the prescribed dose of 1·5mg twice a day is in line with the recommended dose.

◆ *Check* that the drug is available in the same units as the prescription:

The label on the bottle in stock is:

Drug name Rivastigmine

Oral solution

Dose 2mg per millilitre

> Rivastigmine Oral Solution
> 2mg per ml

Having identified that the prescription is in the right range for our patient, and that we have the right drug for the correct route of administration, we can concentrate on the information that is directly relevant to the calculation – the prescribed dose and the strength of the stock preparation.

◆ *Estimate* an approximate answer:

The prescribed amount of 1·5mg is less than 2mg.

As the stock solution is 2mg in 1ml, we need less than 1ml.

◆ *Calculate*

Use your chosen method for calculating:

Method 1: Look for relationships between the numbers involved.

You may recognize that 1·5 is $\frac{3}{4}$ of 2.

So, if there are 2mg in 1ml, there will be 1·5mg in $\frac{3}{4}$ of 1ml.

Required amount = 0·75ml.

75

Method 2: Logic tells you that if there is 2mg in 1ml, then there will be 1mg in $\frac{1}{2}$ml and 0·5mg in half of that ($\frac{1}{4}$ml). So you will need $\frac{1}{2}+\frac{1}{4}$ml = $\frac{3}{4}$ml or 0·75ml.

Method 3: If you know what volume of the liquid contains 1mg of the drug, then you can multiply it by 1·5 to calculate the volume containing 1·5mg.

The label 2mg per ml, tells us that 1mg is in $\frac{1}{2}$ml or 0·5ml.

If 1mg = 0·5ml

Then 1·5mg = 0·5 × 1·5 = 0·75

Required amount is = 0·75ml

Method 4: Apply the formula:

$$\text{Dose} = \frac{\text{what you want}}{\text{what you've got}} \times \frac{\text{what it's in}}{1}$$

Substitute known values:

$$\text{Dose} = \frac{1.5}{2} \times \frac{1}{1}\text{ml}$$

Get rid of the decimal by multiplying top and bottom by 10:

$$= \frac{15}{20} \times 1ml$$

Cancel down by dividing top and bottom by 5:

$$= \frac{3}{4}ml \text{ or } 0.75ml.$$

◆ *Check* that your answer is around the estimated amount and is a sensible amount to be given by the prescribed route.

 ## Practice exercise 5.2 Oral liquid medications with prescription check (suitable for all)

In the examples given below, check that the prescription is within the recommended range prior to calculating the amount of dispensed medication needed for a single dose using the label information supplied.

1 Four-year-old Cameron is feverish and prescribed paracetamol.

Name of drug	Dose	Route	Frequency
PARACETAMOL	200mg	oral	4–6 hrly

Paracetamol: Recommended dose CHILD 1–5 years 120–250mg, 4–6 hrly.

2 Baby Kylie is 2 months old and has just had routine vaccinations.

Name of drug	Dose	Route	Frequency
PARACETAMOL	60mg	oral	6 hrly

Paracetamol: Recommended dose CHILD 2 months 60mg for post-immunization pyrexia. May be repeated 4–6 hrly.

3 Mr Fenn has mild heart failure but cannot swallow tablets.

Name of drug	Dose	Route	Frequency
DIGOXIN	0.25mg	oral	daily

Digoxin: Recommended adult oral dose 125–250 micrograms daily.

4 Six-year-old Paul is allergic to penicillin and has a chest infection.

Name of drug	Dose	Route	Frequency
ERYTHROMYCIN	250mg	oral	6 hrly

Erythromycin: Recommended dose CHILD 2–8 years 250mg every 6 hours.

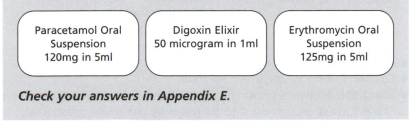

Paracetamol Oral Suspension 120mg in 5ml

Digoxin Elixir 50 microgram in 1ml

Erythromycin Oral Suspension 125mg in 5ml

Check your answers in Appendix E.

Prescriptions based on weight

In neonatal and children's nursing and also when prescribing cytotoxic drugs for cancer, the size of the patient is of paramount importance and doses may differ widely. Checking the prescription as we did above is particularly important when medication is prescribed in relation to a patient's weight. There is an additional calculation to be made when doing this.

Worked example 5.4 Prescription based on weight

A 5-year-old child whose weight is 19kg is to have the antibiotic Amoxicillin orally three times a day for treatment of otitis media.

Date	Name of drug	Dose	Route	Frequency
10/02/08	AMOXICILLIN	250mg	oral	t.d.s.

Remember we now have an *additional stage* for safety in medication calculations, particularly relevant to children or dose by weight, and so our process is as follows.

◆ *Extract* the relevant information from the prescription.

◆ *Check the prescription* especially if unfamiliar with the drug or dealing with children or the elderly.

Use the recommended dose range to check that the prescribed amount is sensible, remembering to take into account the size of the patient, route prescribed and frequency of the dose. (If you are the prescriber, then you will have had to check this from a formulary already.)

◆ *Check* that the drug is available in the same units as the prescription:

Label on the bottle:

> Amoxicillin
> Paediatric Suspension
> 125mg in 1·25ml

◆ *Estimate* an approximate answer.
◆ *Calculate using your chosen method.*
◆ *Check this answer* against the approximation and check that it is a sensible format and amount to be given by the route prescribed.

So let's work this through.

◆ *Extract* the relevant information from the prescription:

The child is prescribed 250mg Amoxicillin orally three times a day.

◆ *Check the prescription*

The British National Formulary (BNF) states that oral Amoxicillin should be prescribed to children with otitis media at a dose of 40 milligram per kilogram (mg/kg) daily, to be given in three divided doses (maximum 3g daily). This information gives us a number of check points: type of infection, dose per weight of the child and the maximum recommended dose. So is the prescription above within the recommended range for our patient?

We need to calculate a number of things:

1 Correct daily dose and whether it is within recommended maximum.

2 Correct divided dose.

3 Amount of drug to give each time based on the available preparation.

1 Correct daily dose for a child of this weight

The child weighs 19kg.

Recommended dose of 40mg per kg tells us that the *daily* dose should be:

$40 \times 19 = 760$mg

Is this within the recommended daily maximum?

Yes, 3g is the recommended daily maximum.

3g = 3000mg and so the amount calculated (760mg) is well within the recommended maximum.

2 The daily dose needs to be divided into three equal doses.

$760 \div 3 = 253$mg

and so each dose should be 253mg.

NB: It would not be sensible to prescribe this exact amount, as it would result in a volume of 2·53ml which is impossible to measure accurately. It is therefore sensible to prescribe a more easily calculated and measured amount.

We can now move on to the next stage:

◆ *Check* that the drug is available in the same units as the prescription.

Amoxicillin is available as:

> Amoxicillin Paediatric
> Suspension 125mg
> in 1·25ml

This is in the same units as the prescription (milligrams).

◆ *Estimate* an approximate answer:

As the prescription is for 250mg, we will need more than the unit dose on the bottle. By approximating the 1·25 to 1, we can see that we will need at least 2ml.

◆ *Calculate using your chosen method*:

Applying the formula: $\dfrac{\textit{what you want}}{\textit{what you've got}} \times \textit{what it's in} = $ dose in ml

Gives us $\dfrac{250}{125} \times \dfrac{1.25}{1} = $ dose in ml

This is a mixture of fractions and decimals and so we need to simplify the fraction. We can do this by cancelling down by dividing top and bottom by 125 or in stages by dividing by 5 or 25, to get:

$2 \times 1\cdot25 = 2\cdot5$ml

◆ *Check this answer* against the approximation and check that it is a sensible format and amount to be given by the route prescribed.

Practice exercise 5.3 Weight-based prescriptions (suitable for adult nurses)

Follow the steps given above for checking the prescription and calculating the dosage for the following patient. Drug labels and prescriptions are shown below.

Mrs Clarke, who weighs 51kg, has been diagnosed with chronic myeloid leukaemia. She has been started on oral Busulfan to induce a remission. The BNF suggests a dose of 60 microgram per kilogram (microgram/kg) to a maximum of 4mg daily.

Name of drug	Dose	Route	Frequency
BUSULFAN	3mg	oral	daily

1 What should be daily dose for Mrs Clarke, based on her weight?

2 Is this prescription within the recommended dose range for Mrs Clarke?

The bottle of tablets carries this label:

> Busulfan Tabs
> 2mg

3 How many tablets should she have?

Unfortunately, the cytotoxic therapy also makes Mrs Clarke feel nauseated and so she is prescribed an anti-emetic, Domperidone. The BNF recommends 10–20mg 3–4 times daily to a maximum of 80mg daily for someone over 34kg.

Name of drug	Dose	Route	Frequency
DOMPERIDONE	15mg	oral	t.d.s.

4 How many anti-emetic tablets are needed for each dose?

> Domperidone
> Tabs
> 10mg

> Domperidone
> Suspension
> 5mg in 5ml

5 As the tablets are not scored, it may be better to give a suspension. How much is needed each dose?

A couple of weeks later, Mrs Clarke appears to be responding to treatment and so the dose of cytotoxic drug is reduced to a maintenance level.

Name of drug	Dose	Route	Frequency
BUSULFAN	1mg	oral	daily

6 How many tablets does she now need to take each day?

Check your answers in Appendix E.

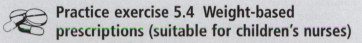

Practice exercise 5.4 Weight-based prescriptions (suitable for children's nurses)

Follow the steps given above for checking the prescription and calculate the dosage for the following patients. For each example, state whether the prescription is safe to give and what amount you would prepare. Drug labels and relevant information from the BNF are shown below.

1 Calum is a young boy weighing 28kg. He is prescribed a diuretic.

Name of drug	Dose	Route	Frequency
FUROSEMIDE	40mg	oral	daily

Furosemide Oral Solution 50mg in 5ml

Furosemide: By mouth, CHILD 1–3mg/kg daily. Maximum 40mg daily.

2 Baby Lucy is 10 weeks old and weighs 7·2kg. She has a very high temperature and is prescribed Paracetamol.

Name of drug	Dose	Route	Frequency
PARACETAMOL	70mg	oral	4–6 hrly (max. 4 doses)

▶

> **Paracetamol Oral Suspension 120mg in 5ml**
>
> *Paracetamol: By mouth, CHILD under 3 months on doctor's advice only, 10mg/kg repeated every 4–6 hours when necessary. Maximum 4 doses in 24 hrs.*

3 Eleven-year-old Hajib weighs 40kg. He has gastric ulceration for which he is prescribed Ranitidine.

Name of drug	Dose	Route	Frequency
RANITIDINE	125mg	oral	8am, 8pm

> **Ranitidine Oral Solution 75mg in 5ml**
>
> *Ranitidine: By mouth, CHILD 2–4mg/kg twice daily. Maximum 300mg daily.*

Check your answers in Appendix E.

 Practice exercise 5.5 Drug calculations (suitable for Mental Health, Adult and Learning Disability nurses)

Follow the steps given above for checking the prescription and calculate the dosage for the following patients. For each example, state whether the prescription is safe to give and what amount you would prepare. Drug labels and relevant information from the BNF are shown below.

Billy Jones is a young man of 19 who has Down's syndrome. He also has an associated heart defect for which he is prescribed a number of drugs. He finds taking tablets very difficult and prefers liquid medicines. He needs help to pour these out accurately. What amount of each of these drugs does he need to take per dose?

	Name of drug	Dose	Route	Frequency
1	DIGOXIN	250 microgram	oral	daily
2	FUROSEMIDE	40mg	oral	daily

Furosemide Oral
Solution
20mg in 5ml

Digoxin Elixir
50 microgram
in 1ml

3 Sharon, aged 11 years, is a friend of Billy and because he has liquid medicines, she wants her medication to be in liquid form too. She has mild epilepsy which causes 'absences'. She is prescribed Zarontin. What volume of medicine should she have per dose?

Name of drug	Dose	Route	Frequency
ZARONTIN (Ethosuximide)	300mg	oral	twice daily

Zarontin Syrup
Ethosuximide
250mg in 5ml

4 This medicine does not suit Sharon. Her weight drops to 35kg and she begins to have fits and so she is prescribed a more effective drug, Sodium Valproate. Check that this is suitable for her weight and calculate the volume required each dose.

Name of drug	Dose	Route	Frequency
SODIUM VALPROATE	350mg	oral	twice daily

Epilim Syrup
Sodium Valproate
200mg in 5ml

Sodium Valproate: By mouth, CHILD over 20kg usual range 20–30mg/kg daily in divided doses. Maximum 35mg/kg daily.

Check your answers in Appendix E.

This chapter has covered prescriptions which take the patient's weight into account. In some cases it is more accurate to calculate a therapeutic dose using the body's surface area as a guide. This is less commonly done and so will be covered in Chapter 8 Further Calculations.

6 Medications Safety: Injections and IV Fluids

This chapter covers:

◆ Routes of injection and sensible volumes (subcutaneous, intramuscular, intravenous, into airway, epidural)

◆ Medication by injection

◆ IV therapy – drip rates for blood and clear fluids using manual sets and volumetric pumps

◆ Syringe drivers

Injections

Medication is given by injection for a number of reasons. It may simply be that the preparation is not suitable for enteral use (via the alimentary tract), the patient may be unable to take the medicine by mouth or it may be that more rapid absorption is required. Nurses and midwives may be required to give or assist with the giving of injections by the following routes:

◆ *intramuscular* – into the muscle, usually outer arm, thigh or buttocks;

◆ *subcutaneous* – into subcutaneous tissue, usually abdomen, outer arm, thigh;

◆ *intradermal* – into the dermis of the skin, usually inner arm, upper back, upper chest;

◆ *intravenous* – directly into a vein;

◆ *epidural* – into the epidural space, via the back;

◆ *intrathecal* – into the cerebro-spinal fluid, via the back;

◆ *via airway* – inhaled into bronchi.

The route of the injection obviously makes a difference to what volume of drug can be given. Injections directly into the blood stream (intravenous) can be of a larger volume than an intramuscular injection; or subcutaneous injection. As an example, if too much anaesthetic is injected into the epidural space, intended to give anaesthesia below the level of injection, it can only disperse upwards and may cause total paralysis and death. Therefore, the nurse has to employ common sense when preparing and/or checking any drug for injection and to recognize what is a sensible amount to give via that particular route. Large amounts injected into muscle or subcutaneously can be very painful.

This is an additional check to be made when calculating the dosage (see Table 6.1). Otherwise, calculating dosage of drugs for injection is just like calculating liquid drug dosages to be given orally.

Table 6.1 Types of injections

Route of injection	Typical volume (in adults)	Example
Intramuscular (IM)	1–3ml	Analgesics, anti-emetics, sedatives, immunizations
Subcutaneous (SC)	0·5–1ml	Heparin and insulin
Intradermal (ID)	Up to 0·5ml	Sensitivity tests, local anaesthetics
Intravenous (IV)	Variable 0–500ml	Antibiotics, analgesia
Epidural	Up to 10ml (block to groin) 15–20ml (block to upper abdomen)	Local anaesthetics/analgesia, opiates
Intrathecal (spinal)	2–4ml	Local anaesthetic/analgesia
Via airway	1–2 puffs	Topical bronchodilators

Just as with oral medicines, you should carry out injection dosage calculations following these stages:

◆ *Extract* the relevant information from the prescription.
◆ *Check the prescription* especially if unfamiliar with the drug or dealing with children or the elderly.
◆ *Check* that the drug is available in the same units as the prescription.
◆ *Estimate* an approximate answer.
◆ *Calculate using your chosen method.*
◆ *Check this answer* against your approximation and check that it is a sensible format and amount to be given by the route prescribed.

Worked example 6.1 Injections

A frail elderly patient is prescribed intramuscular codeine phosphate for relief of pain.

Date	Name of drug	Dose	Route	Frequency
10/02/08	CODEINE PHOSPHATE	45mg	IM	4 times a day

The label on the one millilitre ampoule is:

Codeine Phosphate
60mg/ml

◆ *Extract* the relevant information from the prescription:

We need 45mg of codeine phosphate.

◆ *Check the prescription* especially if unfamiliar with the drug or dealing with children or the elderly:

The BNF information on codeine phosphate advises 30–60mg 4 hourly as necessary, to a maximum of 240mg daily. The prescribed amount of 45mg 4 times a day would result in a total of 4×45mg (180mg) over 24 hours, which is within the daily maximum.

◆ *Check* that the drug is available in the same units as the prescription:

Yes, the prescription is in mg and so is the dispensed product.

◆ *Estimate* an approximate answer:

The required amount is less than the unit dose, but more than half of it and so we need an amount between 0·5 and 1ml.

◆ *Calculate using your chosen method*:

The first two methods are not as easy for this particular dose because there is no obvious relationship between the prescribed dose and the available preparation.

Method 3: If you know what volume of the liquid contains 1mg of the drug, then multiply it by 45 to calculate the volume containing 45mg:

60mg $= 1$ml

Divide both sides of the equation by 60:

therefore 1mg $= \dfrac{1}{60}$ml

and $\qquad 45mg = 45 \times \dfrac{1}{60}ml$

cancel down by dividing top and bottom by 15:

$$= \dfrac{3}{4}ml = 0.75ml$$

Formula: $\dfrac{what\ you\ want}{what\ you've\ got} \times what\ it's\ in = dose$

Substitute from the prescription to get:

$$\dfrac{45}{60} \times \dfrac{1}{1} = \dfrac{45}{60} = \dfrac{3}{4}ml$$

$$= 0.75ml$$

◆ *Check* this answer against your approximation and check that it is a sensible format and amount to be given by the route prescribed.

NB: For optimum accuracy, always use a syringe size as near as possible to the volume of the injection. To draw up 0·75ml, we should use a 1ml syringe if possible (Figure 6.1).

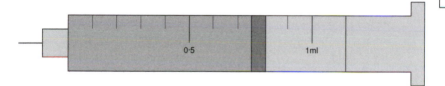

Figure 6.1 A 1ml syringe filled to 0·75ml

Displacement in reconstituted powders

Some injectable drugs are stored as a powder and have to be reconstituted as a liquid before being given. This liquid is usually prescribed or recommended by pharmacy and is termed the **diluent** or, sometimes, **dilutent**. Common diluents are normal saline (0·9% Sodium Chloride) and water for injection. The diluent has to be sterile as does the powder containing the active ingredient of the preparation. Dissolving a powder in a volume of liquid may have the effect of increasing the volume of the liquid as the powder displaces the diluent.

Practice exercise 6.1 Injections (suitable for all)

Calculate the volume to be injected from the prescription excerpts below.

1 This diuretic has been prescribed for Mrs Smith, a well-built lady.

Name of drug	Dose	Route	Frequency
FUROSEMIDE	30mg	IM	daily

2 Joan Darby has a deep-vein thrombosis which is being treated with an anticoagulant.

Name of drug	Dose	Route	Frequency
HEPARIN	15,000 units	SC	twice daily

3 Alf Thomas is breathless following a bee sting.

Name of drug	Dose	Route	Frequency
HYDROCORTISONE	150mg	IM	statim

4 Tony Jones has developed a bone infection following a motor bike accident in which he broke both his legs.

Name of drug	Dose	Route	Frequency
CLINDAMYCIN	300mg	IM	6 hrly

NB: Heparin is an anticoagulant which is measured in active units and comes in several different strengths. Only one label has been illustrated below, but be careful to select the most suitable strength for the dose and route prescribed.

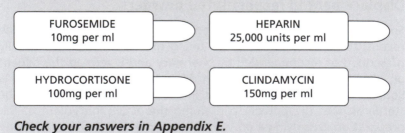

FUROSEMIDE
10mg per ml

HEPARIN
25,000 units per ml

HYDROCORTISONE
100mg per ml

CLINDAMYCIN
150mg per ml

Check your answers in Appendix E.

For example, a prescription for 250mg Amoxicillin, when prepared for intramuscular injection may be reconstituted from powder (250mg) by adding 1·5ml of water for injection (diluent). The result of this reconstitution is 1·7ml of prepared medication. This difference does not matter, except when the reconstituted medicine is not being given in its entirety – when only part of it is required. In this case, it is important to allow for the displacement when calculating the final volume to give. The reconstituted volume may be given in the product literature, or a displacement value may be quoted. In the latter case, this amount must be added to the amount of diluent to give the final volume.

Worked example 6.2 Reconstitution of powdered drug

Amoxicillin prescribed for a 10kg child.

Name of drug	Dose	Route	Frequency
AMOXICILLIN	125mg	IM	6 hrly

Label on vial:

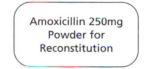

Amoxicillin 250mg
Powder for
Reconstitution

The product literature will inform you of the correct diluent and the displacement value, if any.

Product information preparation instructions for amoxicillin are:

Amoxicillin 250mg Intramuscular injection – add *1·5ml* of *water for injection*. Shake vigorously. Final volume is *1·7ml*.

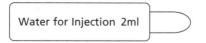

Water for Injection 2ml

◆ *Extract* the required information:

In this case, it is not only the prescription sheet and the labels which are providing information but also the product literature and/or the local pharmacy guidelines.

◆ *Check the prescription*:

The BNF recommendation is as follows:

Intramuscular amoxicillin, CHILD, 50–100mg/kg daily in divided doses.

What is the recommended daily dose for a child of 10kg?

According to this information, it is between 10 × 50mg and 10 × 100mg.

Or 500–1000mg over 24 hours.

What has our patient been prescribed?

125mg given 6 hourly.

This gives a total amount over 24 hours of 4 × 125mg = 500mg.

This is within the recommended range.

◆ *Check* that the drug is available in the same units as the prescription:

Yes, both prescription and preparation are in milligrams.

◆ *Estimate an approximate answer*:

By adding 1·5ml of water to the vial we will have reconstituted 250mg of amoxicillin in 1·7ml.

We need 125mg and so we are going to need half the reconstituted vial.

◆ *Calculate using your chosen method*:

or apply the formula: $\dfrac{\textit{what you want}}{\textit{what you've got}} \times \textit{what it's in} = \text{dose}$

Substitute the known values to get your answer:

$$\frac{\overset{1}{\cancel{125}}}{\underset{2}{\cancel{250}}} \times \frac{1\cdot7}{1} = \frac{1\cdot7}{2}$$

$$= 0\cdot85 \text{ ml}$$

◆ *Check this answer* against your approximation and check that it is a sensible format and amount to be given by the route prescribed.

Practice exercise 6.2 Reconstitution of powdered preparations

Calculate the volume required for the following injections including the checking process for children's dosages where relevant:

1 Amy is a 4-year-old who weighs 16kg. She is prescribed Amoxicillin as shown below.

Name of drug	Dose	Route	Frequency
AMOXICILLIN	400mg	IM	8 hrly

Label on vial:

> Amoxicillin 500mg
> Powder for
> Reconstitution

Intramuscular Amoxicillin, CHILD, 50–100mg/kg daily in divided doses.

Product information preparation instructions are:

Amoxicillin 500mg Intramuscular injection – add 2·5ml of water for injection. Shake vigorously. Final volume is 2·9ml.

Water for Injection 2ml	Water for Injection 2ml

2 Mr Raine has a severe respiratory infection and has been prescribed an intravenous antibiotic.

Name of drug	Dose	Route	Frequency
AUGMENTIN	1·2g	IV	8 hrly

Label on vial:

> Augmentin 600mg
> Powder for
> Reconstitution

Product information preparation instructions:

Co-amoxiclav (*Augmentin*) 600mg dissolved in *10ml of water for injection.*

Water for Injection 10ml

Final volume 10·5ml.

Check your answers in Appendix E.

Intravenous fluids

Intravenous fluids are given to patients for a number of reasons. If patients are unable to take in sufficient fluid orally because of their condition, then they are likely to have all or some of the daily requirement of fluid via an intravenous infusion, often referred to as a 'drip'. Some other reasons for having a 'drip' are in order to receive a blood transfusion, other blood products such as platelets or plasma, potent drugs such as cytotoxic therapy, or intravenous feeding.

In most children's units, intensive care and high tech areas, intravenous fluids are likely to be administered via an electronically controlled volumetric pump. However, you may well come across places which do not have such sophisticated equipment and where a drip rate is just that – the number of drips per minute. This means that you have to calculate that rate from a prescription for intravenous fluids, which might look something like this:

Fluid	Volume	Duration	Start time/date
Dextrose 5%	1 litre	6 hours	13·00 21/01/08

To be able to set up this infusion correctly, you need to know about the equipment available and what it does.

The easiest equipment to use is a volumetric infusion pump, most of which can be used to set the volume to be infused in millilitres and the rate per hour giving a rate of millilitres per hour (ml/hr). This still requires a calculation by the person setting it up to convert the prescribed amount and time into ml/hr.

Worked example 6.3 Volumetric infusion pump

In order to enter the correct information into the pump, we can use the same process as we have used in calculating prescribed medication doses:

◆ *Extract* the relevant information from the prescription for IV fluids above:

The fluid prescribed is 5% Dextrose and the rate is 1 litre over 6 hours.

Is the 5% something which you need to account for in your calculation?

No – in this case, 5% Dextrose is just the name of the fluid prescribed.

◆ *Check* that the drug is available in the same units as the prescription:

This can be interpreted as 'Are the units of the prescription the same units as the delivery device (volumetric pump)?'

No, we have 1 litre of fluid and the pump requires us to enter millilitres.

The prescription time is in hours and we have to enter hours on the pump, so that is OK. So, we need to convert the prescription to the units used by the pump:

1 litre = 1000ml

◆ *Estimate* an approximate answer:

We need to work out what rate 1000ml in 6 hours represents as mls/hr. The rate of anything depends on what it is and the time taken. For example, the rate of a car is the distance it travels divided by the time taken:

$$30 \text{ miles in 1 hour} = \frac{30}{1}\text{mph}$$

$$60 \text{ miles in 2 hours} = \frac{60}{2} = 30\text{mph}$$

The rate of an intravenous infusion is the volume delivered divided by the time taken:

$$Rate = \frac{Volume}{Time}$$

$$1000\text{ml in 6 hours} = \frac{1000}{6}\text{ml/hr}$$

To approximate, it is easier to divide 1000 by 5 which equals 200.

◆ *Calculate*:

$$\frac{\overset{500}{\cancel{1000}}}{\underset{3}{\cancel{6}}} = \frac{500}{3} = 166{\cdot}666\text{ml/hr}$$

◆ *Check* this against estimated rate.

NB: The pump shown allows us to enter a decimal point, but on other pumps we may need to round up or down to the nearest whole number.

◆ *Final check* that you have the correct fluid and the correct volume.

NB: There are other checks which have to be made before setting up an intravenous (IV) infusion but they do not affect the calculation element and so will not be discussed here.

To set the pump, enter 1000 on the pump control panel (Figure 6.2) as the volume to be infused and the rate as close to the calculated value as the device will accept. Some pumps will only allow whole numbers to be entered and so any decimals in the calculated rate need to be rounded (see p. 12 for rounding rules). Pumps used in paediatric units may allow a decimal to be entered. Usually only one decimal place is used and so you need to correct your calculation to one decimal place. In this example we would enter 166·7.

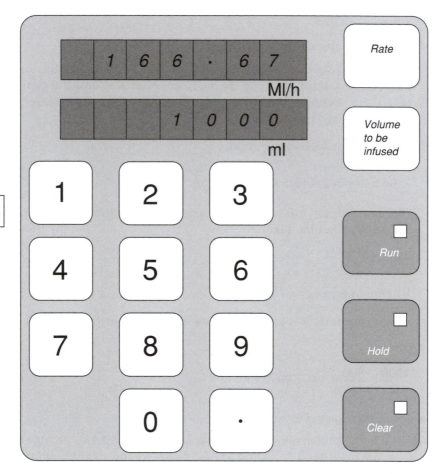

Figure 6.2 A typical volumetric infusion pump control panel

Having set volume and rate, we rely on the electronic pump to deliver the fluid to the patient at the correct rate.

Practice exercise 6.3 Intravenous rates of infusion, volumetric pumps (ml/hr)

Calculate what rate in millilitres per hour you will enter on the volumetric pump for the following fluid prescriptions.

	Fluid	Volume	Duration	Number of decimal places available
1	Dextrose 5%	500ml	3 hours	whole number only
2	Saline 0·9%	1000ml	7 hours	1 decimal place
3	Hartmann's solution	1 litre	4 hours	whole number only
4	Saline 0·9%	500ml	6 hours	1 decimal place
5	Dextrose 10%	1000ml	8 hours	whole number only
6	Sodium Bicarbonate	100ml	45 mins	1 decimal place

Check your answers in Appendix E.

Calculating a manual drip rate

What about a situation where we have not got a volumetric pump? We *could* check the bottle every hour and check that 167mls had gone through, but this would be impossible to estimate given the collapsible nature of most IV fluid containers, so we have to try to set the rate as accurately as possible to start with, by hand.

We can set the drip rate manually by adjusting the roller on the tubing of the intravenous giving set (Figure 6.3) and counting the drops as they enter the drip chamber. To do this, we need to know how to calculate the number of drops to be delivered over a period for which is reasonable to stand there and measure. Hence it is sensible to set a rate of *drops per minute*.

To calculate the number of drops per minute, we need to know the size or volume of each drop, or how many drops there are in a millilitre. The size of the drop delivered by each particular set should be written on the packaging of the IV giving set. A standard set used in many hospitals is one which delivers 20 drops per millilitre for clear fluids but 15 drops per millilitre for blood (proof that blood is thicker than water!). However, it is something that you should check before calculating your drip rate. There are also sets available which

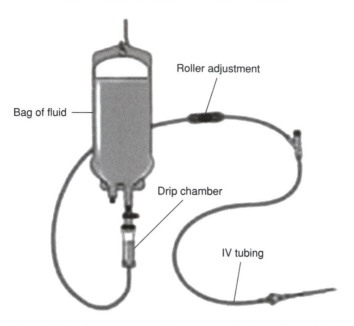

Figure 6.3 An intravenous giving set attached to a bag of fluid

deliver 60 drops per millilitre and can be used in children's nursing, or to give smaller volumes more accurately in adults. These are sometimes referred to as paediatric giving sets.

Worked example 6.4 Manual drip rates

We have already calculated the rate for 1000ml of clear fluid to be delivered over 6 hours using the volumetric pump and we got 166·67ml/hr (correct to two decimal places). To calculate the rate of drops per minute, we need to convert the millilitres into drops and the hours into minutes.

First, let's change the millilitres into drops. Assuming that our giving set delivers 20 drops to a millilitre, 166·67ml will be:

166·67 × 20 drops/1 = 3333·4 drops per hour

Next we need to change the hour into minutes. There are 60 minutes in one hour, so we divide by 60 to get the rate per minute.

Check that this is sensible. At a set rate, an amount delivered over a minute will be less than an amount delivered over an hour and so it is sensible to divide:

3333·4 ÷ 60 = 55·56 drops per minute

We cannot count less than one whole drop, so the obvious thing to do is to round this to the nearest whole number.

Therefore, we need to count 56 drops per minute to get 1 litre delivered in 6 hours.

NB: In practice, and as you become more experienced, timing may be done over 30 or even 15 seconds and so you will actually be counting 56 ÷ 2 (28 drops) or 56 ÷ 4 (14 drops) respectively.

Formula for drop rate

Can we construct a formula for this calculation which will work every time we need to calculate drops per minute from a fluid prescription?

We already have the basic formula:

$$Rate = \frac{Volume}{Time}$$ but this gave us a rate of millilitres per hour.

To get drops per minute, we multiplied the volume in millilitres by the number of drops per ml and divided by 60 to get minutes rather than hours:

$$Rate = \frac{Volume}{Time} \times \frac{drops\ per\ ml}{60}$$

Worked example 6.5 Manual drip rate using formula

Mrs Noon needs a unit of packed blood cells.

Fluid	Volume	Duration	Giving set drop factor
Packed cells	400ml	2 hours	15 drops/ml

Use the formula to calculate the rate at which to set the infusion:

$$Rate = \frac{Volume}{Time} \times \frac{drops\ per\ ml}{60}$$

Substitute the known values in the equation to get:

$$Rate = \frac{400}{2} \times \frac{15}{60}$$

$$= 50 \text{ drops per minute}$$

Worked example 6.6 Drip rate over half an hour

David needs an antibiotic given intravenously over half an hour.

Fluid	Volume	Duration	Giving set drop factor
Vancomycin 500mg	100ml	30 mins	20 drops/ml

$$Rate = \frac{Volume}{Time} \times \frac{drops\ per\ ml}{60}$$

Note that the formula allows for conversion of hours to minutes which we do not need in this case as we already have time in minutes. So the formula becomes:

$$Rate = \frac{Volume}{Time} \times drops\ per\ ml$$

Substitute known values:

$$Rate = \frac{100}{30} \times \frac{20}{1} = \frac{200}{3} = 66{\cdot}66$$

As this number refers to drops, it needs to be rounded up to 67 drops per minute.

Practice exercise 6.4 Manual IV drip rates

Calculate manual drip rates for the following fluid prescriptions taking note of the drop factor information given.

	Fluid	Volume	Duration	Giving set drop factor
1	Dextrose 5%	500ml	5 hours	20 drops/ml
2	Saline 0·9%	1 litre	8 hours	12 drops/ml
3	Hartmann's solution	500ml	6 hours	20 drops/ml
4	Whole blood	500ml	3 hours	15 drops/ml
5	Dextrose 10%	1000ml	12 hours	20 drops/ml
6	Sodium Bicarbonate	100ml	90 mins	60 drops/ml

Check your answers in Appendix E.

Syringe drivers

Particularly in neonates and intensive care environments, intravenous medication may be delivered via a syringe driver where delivery needs to be slower than can be controlled by hand or the amount is too much to give as a **bolus**. Special training is recommended for their use, as incorrect use of syringe drivers is a common cause of drug errors.

As the name suggests, a syringe driver is an electronically controlled device which pushes the plunger of a horizontal syringe at a constant set rate. It allows constant delivery of small amounts over a set period of time. Rate of delivery depends on the type of device and normally the calculation required for the rate is for millilitres per hour. However, some devices are designed to allow the plunger to move a measured distance over time and so deliver the content contained within *millimetres* of syringe length per unit of time, rather than volume. The nurse needs to measure the length of the fluid column in the syringe in order to set the correct rate. This will of course depend on the size and make of syringe and requires a great deal of care to ensure correct dosages are given.

In most hospital units, electronic syringe drivers are used which, with the correct syringe inserted, can be programmed to deliver millilitres per hour. The examples given here will refer to this type of device. Syringe drivers may be used for constant delivery of a drug or for intermittent delivery at intervals.

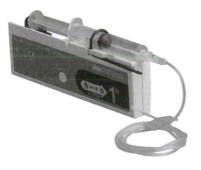

Figure 6.4 Example of a portable syringe driver using length (mm) of fluid in syringe per hour as the measurement of rate of delivery

Worked example 6.7 Syringe driver rates

An adult prescription for endocarditis, a severe infection of the heart lining, is:

Name of drug	Dose	Route	Frequency
AMOXICILLIN	2g	IV	6 hourly

◆ *Extract* the required information from the prescription sheet, the labels and the product literature and/or the local pharmacy guidelines:

Label on vial:

> Amoxicillin 1g
> Powder for
> Reconstitution

Label on ampoule:

> Water for Injection 20ml

The product literature/pharmacy guidelines suggest reconstitution as follows:

Amoxicillin for IV infusion – give over 30 minutes to 1 hour.

Add 20ml water for injection to 1g powder, final volume 20·8ml.

◆ *Check* that the drug is available in the same units as the prescription:

Both prescription and preparation are in gram.

◆ *Estimate* an approximate answer:

By adding 20ml of water to the vial we will have reconstituted 1g of amoxicillin. We need 2g and so we are going to have to use 2 vials and 2 ampoules of water and so it will be approximately 40ml.

◆ *Calculate using your chosen method*:

This one is quite straightforward. By reconstituting as directed, we will get:

1g in 20·8ml and

2g in 2 × 20·8ml = 41·6ml

◆ *Check this answer* against the approximation and check that it is a sensible format and amount to be given by the route prescribed:

Now we have to set the syringe driver to deliver the drug at an appropriate rate. This is a case of intermittent delivery (every 6 hours) but over 30 minutes to an hour. As the volume we have calculated is nearly 42ml, it would be appropriate to set the syringe driver to 42ml/hour.

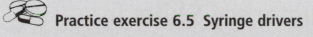 **Practice exercise 6.5 Syringe drivers**

Check the prescriptions below and calculate the volume of drug to be given and the rate of the syringe driver in mls per hour.

1 Sophie weighs 25kg and has been ordered intravenous antibiotics.

Name of drug	Dose	Route	Frequency
GENTAMYCIN	50mg	IV infusion	t.d.s. given over 30 mins

Gentamicin CHILD 2mg/kg 8 hrly

Label on vial:

> Gentamycin
> In Sodium Chloride
> For IV Infusion
> 800 micrograms
> in 1ml

2 Mrs Moss has advanced cancer and is being given relief from nausea via a subcutaneous infusion as she cannot manage oral medication.

Name of drug	Dose	Route	Frequency
HALOPERIDOL	7·5mg	SC infusion	over 24 hours

Label on ampoule: Haloperidol 5mg per ml

Check your answers in Appendix E.

This chapter has covered common calculations related to injections and IV fluids. The next chapter will look at the types of calculations you may come across when monitoring patients' fluid balance.

7 Numeracy Skills in Fluid Balance

This chapter covers:

◆ **General fluid balance**

◆ **Special cases** – irrigation and dialysis

◆ **Fluid balance in children**

Calculations related to fluid balance are usually very straightforward, as they require only addition and subtraction. However, other uses of numeracy come into play when looking at fluid balance and the nurse and midwife also need to have an understanding of measures associated with weight, volume and time. In children's nursing and when nursing neonates, the calculations can become more complicated.

The chapter will begin by looking at fluid balance calculations used in adult nursing and then progress to the more difficult calculations required for specialist situations.

In health, the body maintains a dynamic balance between fluid and electrolyte intake and loss. A 24-hour period (1 day) is considered as a suitable time period over which a balance should be maintained. In other words, the amount of fluid taken in over 24 hours should equal the amount being lost, by all routes. There are many conditions which affect the individual's ability to maintain this balance, both physical and psychological and, as a nurse or midwife you are almost certain to come across patients/clients in whom the balance is upset. Maintaining fluid balance is therefore a common component of nursing duties and a very important one.

Minimal fluid requirements vary from person to person depending on their size and level of activity and standardized tables are available. Patients in hospital may have specific needs and so their requirements can differ from those published. For example, if a patient is already dehydrated, then they will need more fluid than the standard stated requirement and the aim will be to end up in a positive balance at the end of the day. Obviously this situation would require monitoring and would need a comparison of daily 'balances' over a number of days. Similarly, in a patient who has accumulated fluid overload, perhaps because of heart failure, the nurse will be looking for a negative balance at the end of the day. This will indicate how effective therapy such as medication with diuretics has been. Normal maintenance daily fluid requirements for an adult are approximately 1ml/kg/hr. This amount would be increased in fever and to account for losses such as wound drainage.

Fluid balance charts

Different establishments use different charts and methods for monitoring fluid balance will differ depending on how the chart is used. The chart may start and finish at 07.00 hrs, allowing the next day's fluid requirements to be set first thing in the morning. Other establishments use charts which start and finish around midnight, arguing that the least activity to do with fluid intake and output in most patients is at this time and so it is a sensible time to do the totting up. It also means that the chart needs to be dated only once. Other differences may be in how the amounts are totalled and when the balance calculation is made. For example, there may be a column which allows for a running total of both input and output and running balance, or the chart may be balanced only once a day. Considering the body's responses to fluids, a daily balance is generally adequate. However, in a patient who has poor renal function, is losing significant amounts of blood or other body fluids or has a brain injury which prevents the normal homeostatic processes occurring, a more frequent recording of balance may be required. Some units/wards require IV fluids to be added in only on completion, others add them in when they are put up and subtract the amount remaining at the end of the calculation period. It is important that you understand the process used where you are working, as errors can be made through different interpretations of the same data being made. Accurately kept fluid balance charts can be very informative.

Worked example 7.1 Fluid balance chart (FBC)

Look at Figure 7.1 which is a fluid balance chart for John Smith, who weighs 73kg. There are several things to do with the numbers on the chart which you should notice and that require you to apply your nursing knowledge. The numbers can tell us more than just the fluid balance, they can help us plan care. Volumes are all in millilitres, but this is not indicated on the chart which is common practice.

ESSENTIAL CALCULATION SKILLS

Name: John Smith					Hospital No. 1234567		Date: Friday 7th March 2008				
Time	Oral	Intravenous 1	Intravenous 2	Intravenous 3	Other	Total IN	Urine	Vomit	Other	Total OUT	Balance -ve/+ve
0100		Dext 5% 100									
0200		N.Saline (1000)				100					+100
0300											
0400											
0500											
0600											
0700	120					120					+120
0800	50					50	320		Drain 100 red	420	-370
0900								100		100	-100
1000		Dext 5% (1000)				1000					+1000
1100	100					100					+100
1200							150			150	-150
1300	200					200					+200
1400	50					50					+50
1500							200	140		340	- 340
1600	180					180			Drain 50 pink	50	+130
1700											
1800	50	N.Saline (1000)				1050	270			270	+780
1900								100			-100
2000	100					100					+100
2100											
2200	150					150	230		Drain 10 clear	240	-90
2300											
2400		N.Saline 850				850					+850
Total	1000	2950				3950	1170	340	160	1670	+2280
Daily Total						3950			+800 =	2470	+1480

Figure 7.1 Fluid balance chart
Note: Based on that used by Royal Wolverhampton Hospitals NHS Trust with their permission.

First of all, note how the balance for the 24-hour period has been calculated. Because the amounts are totalled both by *row* and by *column*, we have an automatic check on the accuracy of our calculations. Notice that the numbers have been kept neatly so that accurate adding and subtraction is easier. Totalling fluid balance charts is a situation where it is sensible to check your calculations using a calculator. Because there are inbuilt checking mechanisms through the row and column totals mentioned above, use of a calculator may make the task quicker.

Notice how the intravenous fluids on this chart have not been added in to the input total until the patient has actually received them but the amount 'put up' is in brackets. There is an entry at the beginning of the chart of 100ml Dextrose 5%. This appears as the amount left to be infused when the previous day's chart ended at midnight. Notice how the final total for intravenous fluids on this chart includes the portion of the current infusion which has already been infused. The remainder will be entered on the next day's chart.

In the final row of the chart you will see that the amount +800 is printed on the chart to be added to the total output. This is a figure representing the insensible loss of fluid which occurs through expiration, evaporation of sweat and fluid content of normal faeces.

What sort of things might this chart indicate to us?

◆ Look at the intake which is about the recommended amount for his weight. If a patient is able to drink as normally as this suggests, then the IV fluids may be unnecessary.

◆ Look at the output. Urine output is not abnormal but it is less than would be expected from the amount of intake. It may be that Mr Smith was slightly dehydrated and is compensating. It would be worth checking the previous day's chart.

◆ The amount of wound drainage is tailing off. This might indicate that it is time for the drain to be shortened or removed.

◆ If you look carefully, you may also notice that the patient appears to vomit a small amount after having had an oral intake amount entered as 50ml. This might suggest that the small amount is taken with some oral medication and that the vomiting might be associated with this. He does not appear to vomit after meals or other drinks. This is something worth mentioning and investigating as his medication may need to be changed.

While this textbook does not cover nursing care *per se*, this is an illustration of how much you can learn from numbers and how important it is to calculate correctly and to keep accurate records.

Practice exercise 7.1 Fluid balance chart (i)

Use the fluid balance chart provided for Mrs Julie Beaver in Figure 7.2 and fill in the total for each row before calculating the final fluid balance for 24 hours. Then check your calculations by totalling the columns.

1 Total input.
2 Total output.
3 24-hour balance.

Name: Julir Beaver	Oral			Hospital No. 9876543			Date: Friday 7th March 2008				
Time	Oral	Intravenous 1	Intravenous 2	Intravenous 3	Other	Total	Urine	Vomit	Other Drain	Total	Balance -ve/+ve
0100		N.Saline 760	Blood 100						150 (blood)		
0200											
0300							100	90			
0400			Discontinued								
0500											
0600	10	5% Dext. 1000					150				
0700	10										
0800	10							60	100		
0900											
1000	80						350				
1100											
1200	90								50 red		
1300							400				
1400	100	1000 Dextrose saline									
1500											
1600	100										
1700											
1800	120						300		20		
1900											
2000		IV Discontinued 300 ml discarded									
2100	180										
2200							350				
2300											
2400											
Total											
Daily Total									+800 =		

Figure 7.2 Fluid balance chart for Practice Exercise 7.1

Check your answers in Appendix E.

Some patients are given fluid which is expected to be returned, for example, as bladder irrigation or peritoneal dialysis fluid. This may be entered on a separate chart or may be integral within the normal fluid balance chart. The calculation of fluid balance for such patients requires keeping a careful record of just how much fluid is being exchanged.

Worked example 7.2 FBC including irrigation fluid

Robert Vale is a 60-year-old man who has had a transurethral prostatectomy and requires continuous bladder irrigation. As you can see, the normal fluid balance chart (FBC) has been adapted for his case. An extract from it is shown below.

Name: Robin Vale				Hospital No. 2468102			Date: Friday 7th March 2008				
Time	Oral	Intravenous 1	Intravenous 2	~~Intravenous~~ ⊖ Irrigation	Other	Total	Urine	Vomit	Other Bladder Drain	Total	Balance -ve/+ve
0800	120	5% Dext 100		N.Saline 250		490			600 br.red	600	
0900		IV Disc									
1000	100			N.Saline 1000		350			600 red	600	
1100	180					180					
1200	200					200			500 clear pk	500	

The final totals for the day were:

Total	2100	100		3750		5950			5150		
Daily Total						5950			+800=	5950	0

The calculations are the same as for any other fluid balance chart, we need to add up the total amount going in and subtract the amount coming out, not forgetting to allow for insensible losses. Notice that as with the IV fluids in the earlier examples of fluid balance charts, the irrigation fluid has not been recorded in the total column until it has all gone in.

The difference here is that we can only account for urine output by looking at the difference in totals between the column headed 'irrigation' and that headed 'bladder drainage'. In this example, the amount of irrigation fluid used was 3750mls and the bladder drainage was 5150. Therefore urine output must have been the total bladder drainage *minus* the amount of irrigation fluid. In other words:

5150 − 3750 = 1400ml.

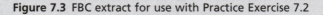

Practice exercise 7.2 Fluid balance chart (ii)

Using the 12-hour extract from a fluid balance chart for Joseph Murphy, illustrated in Figure 7.3, calculate the following.

1 Joseph's total intake (use row/column totals to check your answer).

2 His total output (use row/column totals to check your answer).

3 His fluid balance at the end of the 12-hour period.

4 The actual urine output.

Name: *Joseph murphy*				Hospital No. 9876543			Date: Friday 7th March 2008				
Time	Oral	Intravenous 1	Intravenous 2	~~Intravenous~~ & Irrigation	Other	Total	Urine	Vomit	Other Bladder Drain	Total	Balance -ve/+ve
0800	180	550 0.9% Saline					25				
0900											
1000	50			N. Saline 1000					620 red		
1100	120										
1200		IV Disc							750 red		
1300	200										
1400									dark pink 555		
1500											
1600	180			N.Saline 1000					580 pink		
1700											
1800	530								650 rose		
1900											
2000	180								670 pale rose		
Total											

Figure 7.3 FBC extract for use with Practice Exercise 7.2

Check your answers in Appendix E.

Dialysis

In order to stay alive, patients in severe renal failure need to have their kidney function replaced by some other means. This artificial process of 'cleansing' the blood is called **dialysis**. *Haemo-dialysis* works on the principle of taking the patient's blood out of the body and circulating it across a membrane where unwanted elements are extracted by osmosis/diffusion and withdrawn from the blood while required substances are retained and/or can be added. The blood is then reintroduced to the body. *Haemofiltration* is another method of managing renal failure in which a semi-permeable membrane allows a filtrate of plasma to be excreted and the losses are replaced by intravenous solutions. An alternative is *peritoneal dialysis*, a process involving the introduction of dialysis fluid into the peritoneum where the body's own capacity for osmosis will exchange electrolytes which are lacking for those products which the body needs to excrete. The fluid itself is the transport medium for the waste products and so it is essential to keep an accurate record of just how much goes in and how much comes out as well as keeping a normal fluid balance record for these patients. Sometimes the patient, particularly in paediatrics, is nursed on a weigh bed which allows for constant monitoring of their weight, which is an additional check of how much fluid is being lost or retained.

Worked example 7.3 Peritoneal dialysis

Mrs Lake has begun continuous peritoneal dialysis and her weight is being recorded hourly, along with a record of the fluid balance relating to her dialysis. An extract from her chart is shown below. Note that the cumulative total is a running total of the amount of fluid lost or gained at the time of entry.

Weight (kg)	Solution IN (fill time 10 min)			Solution OUT (drain time 20 min)			Difference per cycle	Cumulative difference (ml)
	Start	Finish	Vol (ml)	Start	Finish	Vol (ml)		
51·5	09·00	09·10	2000	10·00	10·20	2100	−100	−100
51·25	10·20	10·30	2000	11·30	11·50	1950	+50	−50
51·67	11·50	12·00	2000	13·00	13·20	1830	+170	+120
51·61	13·20	13·30	2000	14·30	14·50	2150	−150	−30
50·4	14·50	15·00	2000	16·00	16·20	2300	−300	−330
51·45	16·20	16·30	2000	17·30	17·50	1740	+260	−70
							Sub-total	−70

By recording the loss or gain at each cycle and totalling this column, we have an instant check of our cumulative total.

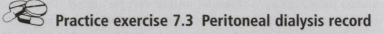

Practice exercise 7.3 Peritoneal dialysis record

1 Use the dialysis record shown below to calculate the cumulative difference in fluid levels between 8am and 12 midday.

Weight (kg)	Solution IN (fill time 10 min)			Solution OUT (drain time 20 min)		
	Start	Finish	Vol (ml)	Start	Finish	Vol (ml)
60·49	08·00	08·10	2000	09·00	09·20	2150
60·43	09·20	09·30	2000	10·20	10·40	2010
60·51	10·40	10·50	2000	11·40	12·00	1895

2 What is the recorded difference in the patient's weight over this period?

Check your answers in Appendix E.

Infant fluids

Babies and young children are more at risk from fluid imbalance due to immature kidneys and being less able to help themselves to fluid when thirsty. Newborn babies need about 150ml per kg of body weight per day. This means that the total amount calculated then needs to be divided by 6 or 8 in order to give 4 or 3 hourly feeds as required. In maternity and children's hospitals in the UK this will probably be calculated by the dietician and sent up from the milk kitchen ready prepared. However, as the person giving the feed, you must be sure that the amount is correct for the individual baby.

Worked example 7.4 Infant feeds

How much feed would you expect to be giving to a 3·28kg baby aged one week? First, calculate the recommended daily amount for the baby:

150ml per kg of body weight is

$150 \times 3.28 = 492$ml

For 4 hourly feeds, divide by 6:

$492 \div 6 = 82$ml per feed

For 3 hourly feeds, divide by 8:

$492 \div 8 = 61\cdot5$ml per feed

Then check – is this what has been prepared and is it a sensible amount for the size of baby?

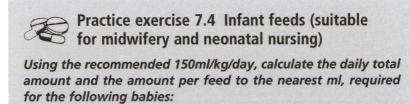

Practice exercise 7.4 Infant feeds (suitable for midwifery and neonatal nursing)

Using the recommended 150ml/kg/day, calculate the daily total amount and the amount per feed to the nearest ml, required for the following babies:

1 Mahmood, weight 2·41kg and on 2 hourly feeds.
2 Jilly, weight 4·15kg, on 4 hourly feeds.
3 Sophie, weight 3·76kg, on 3 hourly feeds.

Check your answers in Appendix E.

Infant feeds and fluid balance

Children require fluid input in volume related to their weight. Correct calculation of fluid balance is particularly vital in children, especially those with cardiac, renal or liver function problems who may have restricted intake. Pre-term babies and those receiving phototherapy may require additional fluids and enterally fed infants will often require higher fluid allowance for optimal growth. Feeds have to be taken into account and *all* fluid measured, including drug volumes.

The type of calculation, which the nurse may need to make, is to work out what volume of maintenance feed (fluid containing nutrients) can be given within the total fluid allowance. This allows the dietician to make up the content appropriately. There may be slight variations in local guidelines for recommended ml/hr/kg. Typical amounts are shown in Table 7.1. The calculation may involve percentages, addition and subtraction.

Neat charts make addition of columns much easier and reduce the risk of calculation errors. Using your calculator to add up totals is fine, but you need to cross-check regularly to a running total.

Table 7.1 Maintenance of intravenous fluid requirements

Weight (kg)	100% Maintenance ml/hour
3	12
4	16
6	24
8	32
10	40
12	45
14	50
16	55
18	60
20	65
30	70
40	80
50	90
60	95
>70	100

Note: Reproduced with kind permission from Birmingham Children's Hospital NHS Trust.

Table 7.1 is intended to be used to calculate appropriate fluid requirements. Fluids should be prescribed as a percentage of normal maintenance rather than ml/kg. That is: a child weighing 40kg being restricted to 50% of normal should receive 40ml/hr. Pre-term babies and those receiving phototherapy may require additional fluids. Enterally fed infants will often require a higher fluid allowance for optimum growth (up to 150% of values given in Table 7.1).

Different NHS Trusts use different proformas, but the nurse needs to be aware of how to fill these in using the local conventions.

Worked example 7.5 Bolus feeds

A 6-month-old infant weighing 6·7kg is to have 5 bottle feeds a day. She also has a combination of intravenous (IV) drugs prescribed, which amount to 12·5ml every 6 hours. How much feed can she have per bottle?

First, calculate the recommended daily amount of fluid for a baby of this weight:

150ml per kg of body weight = 150 × 6·7 = 1005ml

Next, calculate how much fluid she is receiving in IV drugs per day:

12·5ml every 6 hours is the same as 4 × 12·5ml over 24 hours = 4 × 12·5 = 50ml

Subtract the total volume of drugs from the fluid allowance to get the remainder which can be given as feed:

$$1005 - 50 = 955ml$$

For the amount per feed, divide this by number of feeds per day (5):

$$955 \div 5 = 191ml$$

This is approximately 190ml per bottle. *Check*: is this a sensible amount for a baby's bottle feed?

Worked example 7.6 Continuous feeding

A child weighing 12kg is prescribed 75% of maintenance fluids over 24 hours. He is being fed continuously by a naso-gastric tube attached to a feed pump. Approximately, how much of the hourly intake should be fed?

According to local policy, 100% maintenance intravenous fluid requirements for a 12kg child is 45ml/hour (see Table 7.1). So what is 75% of 45ml/hr?

◆ First, do a rough *estimate*:

75% is the same as $\frac{3}{4}$ so the amount must be less than 45 (the whole amount) but more than 22 (approximately half):

$$75\% = \frac{75}{100}$$

$$75\% \text{ of } 45 = \frac{75}{100} \times 45ml/hr$$

divide top and bottom by 25 to give $\frac{75^3}{100_4} \times \frac{45}{1}$

then multiply across to get $\frac{135}{4}$

Use the percentage key on your calculator instead of dividing by 100 if you wish, but always check your answer against the estimate.

The answer is 33·75. So the child should be receiving a total of 33·75ml per hour.

But when you look at the prescription sheet, you realize that continuous infusions of various drugs amount to 5ml/hour and antibiotics add another 15ml every 6 hours. Taking these into account, what is the amount of feed which can be given per hour?

◆ First, *calculate* the total volume of prescribed drugs/fluid per hour:

IV infusions = 5ml/hour

Antibiotics = 15ml in 6 hours = 15 ÷ 6 = 2·5ml/hr

Total volume of infusions/drugs per hour is 7·5ml

Therefore, the child can be given a feed of

$$\begin{array}{r} 3\ 3\ \cdot\ 7\ 5 \\ 7\ \cdot\ 5\quad - \\ \hline 2\ 6\ \cdot\ 2\ 5 \ \ \text{ml/hr} \end{array}$$

◆ *Check* that this is a sensible amount.

Practice exercise 7.5 High dependency infant fluids

Where required, use Table 7.1, Maintenance of Intravenous Fluid Requirements to help work out the following:

Chloe, aged 10 days and weighing 3kg is receiving 3·5ml/hr via IV infusion and 8·8ml of drugs 6 hourly. She is on 100% maintenance volume.

1 What is 100% maintenance over 24 hours for Chloe?

2 What volume per 24 hours is she getting by IV infusion?

3 How much do her drugs contribute?

4 How much feed can she be given over the 24-hour period?

Chloe has been operated on for a minor heart defect and is now 1 day post-operation. She is now allowed only 40% maintenance volume and her drugs have been changed to 5·5ml 3 hourly. Her intravenous infusion is running at 1ml/hour.

5 What is 40% maintenance over 24 hours?

6 How much is she getting via the IV?

7 What volume of drugs is given in 24 hours?

8 What is the total volume of feed she can have?

Chloe is making good progress and is now allowed 60% maintenance fluids. The total volume of drugs and IV fluids remains the same.

9 What is 60% maintenance?

10 What is the new volume of feed permitted?

By the end of the third post-operative day, Chloe's drugs have been reduced to 4·8ml 6 hourly, her intravenous fluids have been stopped and she can have 100% of her maintenance fluid allowance made up as feed.

11 How much fluid volume does her new drug regime entail over 24 hrs?

12 What volume of feed is she now allowed?

Check your answers in Appendix E.

We have now seen how to deal with the common types of calculations you are likely to encounter in general situations. As pointed out, there are some areas of nursing such as in intensive care and in high dependency units, where more complicated calculations are required. The next chapter is intended to cover the more common calculations you may come across in these specialist areas.

8 Further Calculations

This chapter covers:

♦ Calculations involving percentages and ratios
♦ Complex prescriptions
♦ Use of nomograms
♦ Neonates/PICU
♦ Calculations based on body surface area (BSA)

Percentages and ratios

The concepts of percentage and ratio were covered briefly in Chapter 2, but actually using them in calculations can be a source of anxiety. The calculations themselves are not difficult, but many people have trouble in understanding what the numbers mean and so can make errors relating to magnitude, which may be very dangerous. When doing calculations involving percentages, ratios or proportion, the golden rule of estimation should always be applied.

Percentage solutions used in healthcare generally indicate grams of solid dissolved in 100ml of solution. A commonly used intravenous fluid is 5% Dextrose. Remember that percentage means 'in a hundred' and 5% is the same as $\frac{5}{100}$.

So, the 5% in *5% Dextrose* indicates that in every 100ml of the solution, there are 5 grams of dextrose, since by scientific convention; 1ml water is equivalent to 1g.

Worked example 8.1 Percentage (i)

We want to know how much dextrose is in a litre (1000ml) bag of 5% dextrose. In other words, what is 5% of 1000ml?

$$\frac{1000}{1} \times \frac{5}{100}$$

We can simplify by dividing top and bottom by 100 to get:

$10 \times 5 = 50g$.

Thus, there is 50g dextrose in a litre bag of 5% Dextrose.

Expressing fractions as percentages and vice versa

To express a fraction as a percentage, multiply by 100. Thus, $\frac{1}{2}$ expressed as a percentage is $\frac{100}{2}$ or 50%.

And to express a percentage as a fraction or decimal, divide by 100. Thus, 25% is the same as $\frac{25}{100}$ which simplifies to $\frac{1}{4}$ or 0·25.

Worked example 8.2 Percentage (ii)

A local anaesthetic cream contains 2·5% lidocaine. How much lidocaine is there in a 5 gram tube? In other words, what is 2·5% of 5?

Calculate: $\dfrac{2\cdot5}{100} \times \dfrac{5}{1}$

Multiply across the fraction to get $\frac{12\cdot5}{100}$ and then divide by 100 by moving the decimal point

$= 0\cdot125g$

So a 5g tube of the cream contains 0·125g of lidocaine.

Worked example 8.3 Percentage (iii)

Chlorhexidine 0·05% can be used for cleansing wounds. What is the strength of this solution in mg/ml?

We know that percentage solutions used in healthcare indicate grams of solid dissolved in 100ml of solution and so 0·05% indicates 0·05g in 100ml. If 100ml = 0·05g (it will be easier to change this to 50mg at this point), then:

$1ml = \dfrac{50}{100}mg = 0\cdot5mg$

So, the strength of a 0·05% solution is 0·5mg/ml.

Worked example 8.4 Percentage (iv)

Percentages are often used in reports. For example, the rate of home births in a region may be reported as 4%. This means that for every hundred births recorded in the region, 4 will have been home deliveries.

A local authority reports a Caesarean section (CS) rate of 24% of births in 2007. If the total number of births under that authority in 2007 was 30,642, how many were delivered by CS? The calculation is:

24% of 30,642

$$\frac{24}{100} \times 30{,}642$$

With numbers as big as this, it is easiest to simplify first before multiplying across:

$$= 24 \times 306{\cdot}42$$
$$= 7354{\cdot}08$$

As this number applies to births, we can sensibly disregard the ·08 and conclude that there were 7354 Caesarean sections in this local authority in 2007.

Worked example 8.5 Percentage (v)

We could equally work out the percentage rate if we knew the total number of deliveries and the number which were Caesarean sections. Thus, 5000 CS deliveries in a total of 31,500 deliveries would mean a percentage rate of:

$$\frac{5000}{31{,}500} \times \frac{100}{1}\,\% = 15{\cdot}9\%$$

Practice exercise 8.1 Percentages

Express the following as a percentage:

1 $\frac{2}{5}$ 　　　　　3 0·8

2 $\frac{3}{50}$ 　　　　　4 0·01

Express the following as a decimal:

5 70% 　　　　　6 12·5%

Calculate:

7 25% of 84 　　　8 10% of 500

9 How much glucose is there in 200ml of 10% glucose solution?

10 What is the strength (mg/ml) of 0·5% lidocaine?

11 What is the percentage of home births in local authority Y where total births number 50,202 and 1578 were born at home?

12 If 1 in three adults on a particular anti-epileptic drug experience visual defects, what is this as a percentage?

Check your answers in Appendix E.

Ratios and proportion

One source of confusion and potential error in medication calculations relates to the use of solutions whose strength is given as a proportion or ratio. Common examples are wound dressings and skin preparations such as Potassium permanganate 1 in 1000.

In order to understand the strength of a solution, we should be able to recognize what this means. 1 in 1000 is the same as $\frac{1}{1000}$ or 0·1%, which means one part of active ingredient in 1000 parts of the solution.

To convert a percentage to a proportion, change it into a fraction first.

Worked example 8.5 Proportions

What is a 0·02% solution as a proportion?

We need to express it as a fraction with a whole number on the top:

$$0·02\% = \frac{0·02}{100}$$

to convert the 0·02 to a whole number, we multiply by 100. So that we do not change the value of the fraction, we do the same to the denominator, resulting in:

$$\frac{2}{10,000} \text{ or, when simplified, } \frac{1}{5000}$$

so we can say that a 0·02% solution is the same as 1 in 5000 solution.

Many things which require dilution, such as milk powders, have specific instructions as to the number of measures of powder to liquid and so are easy to calculate. However, the final result should always be checked to see if it is sensible.

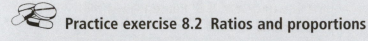

Practice exercise 8.2 Ratios and proportions

1 How would you express 1 in 50 as a percentage?

2 Express 0·01% as a proportion.

3 What is 1 in 2000 as a percentage?

4 What is 0·5% as a proportion?

5 Express 1 in 5000 as a percentage.

Check your answers in Appendix E.

Worked example 8.6 Dilution of solutions

Potassium permanganate is available as a 0·1% or 1 in 1000 solution, but for use as a wet dressing, the BNF suggests further dilution with water to 1 in 10,000.

Let us suppose that we need 100ml of solution.

◆ *Estimate* – the required solution is 10 times weaker than the stock available, and so we are going to need a tenth of the stock solution. In 100ml, this would be 10ml. By estimating, we can see that we do not actually need to do a calculation, but the calculation needed will be included to illustrate the principle.

◆ Then, *calculate* how much active ingredient would be in 100ml of the required solution which is 1 in 10,000.

1 in 10,000 = 0·01%

This means 0·01g in 100ml, and so we require 0·01g of active ingredient. To get this amount from the stock solution (0·1% or 0·1g in 100ml), we can use the methods of dosage calculation used throughout the book.

◆ *Applying the formula*:

$$\text{Dose} = \frac{\textit{what you want}}{\textit{what you've got}} \times \frac{\textit{what it's in}}{1}$$

And substituting values, we get:

$$\frac{0\cdot01}{0\cdot1} \times \frac{100}{1}\text{ml} = 10\text{ml}$$

So, we require 10ml of the stock solution and 90ml of water to produce the required strength.

Practice exercise 8.3 Percentages and proportions

1 What is the amount of active ingredient in 10ml of a 1 in 10,000 solution?

2 A 1% solution is required but the only available strength is 10%. How much of this will be required to produce 50ml of 1% solution and how much diluent?

3 An epidural infusion of Bupivacaine 0·1% is required during labour. How much 0·25% solution and how much diluent will you need to make up 60ml of the required strength?

4 During a resuscitation procedure, 8ml of an ampoule of adrenaline 1 in 10,000 was given to the patient. How much adrenaline did he receive?

Check your answers in Appendix E.

Complex prescriptions

Patients requiring intensive care are often on a variety of drugs which are part of a life support system. The calculations required to ensure that correct dosages are received can be quite difficult as they can involve several different measurements including the patient's weight, strength of solution and rate of delivery. Inotropic drugs which are used to increase the force of cardiac contraction are a good example of this. Because of their potency, they are generally administered via a central venous line rather than a peripheral line and delivery is always controlled through a delivery device such as an electronic syringe pump/driver.

121

Worked example 8.7 Complex prescriptions

An adult male weighing 80kg requires dobutamine at a rate of 5 microgram/kg/min.

Name of drug	Amount	Route	Frequency
DOBUTAMINE	Solution made up in Dextrose 5% as 3mg/kg in total volume of 50ml	IV via central line	5ml/hr

Recommended adult dose is 2 microgram/kg/min – 10 microgram/kg/min.

Label on ampoule:

> Dobutamine
> 250mg in 20ml

◆ *Extract* the relevant information from the prescription:

Drug = 3mg/kg Dobutamine

The diluent is 5% Dextrose. (Note that the 5% is just a part of the labelling and does not come into the calculation.)

◆ *Check the prescription.*

The rate prescribed is within the recommended guidelines.

If made up as directed, how much Dobutamine is needed and will this give the correct amount for our patient?

Stage 1: Make up solution

◆ *Check* that the drug is available in the same units as the prescription:

Yes, both are milligrams.

◆ *Estimate dose*:

Weight 80kg × 3mg = 240mg Dobutamine

Dobutamine comes as 250mg in a 20ml ampoule

240mg is nearly 250 and so we will need just under 20ml.

◆ *Calculate using your chosen method:*

Apply the formula: $\dfrac{\textit{what you want}}{\textit{what you've got}} \times$ *what it's in* = dose

Substitute the known values to get your answer:

$$\frac{240}{250} \times \frac{20}{1} = \frac{96}{5}$$

$$= 19{\cdot}2\text{ml}$$

◆ *Check this answer* against your approximation.

To make up the required solution to a total of 50ml, we have to add (50 − 19·2)ml of diluent. We will use 5% Dextrose:

= 30·8 Dextrose 5%

We now have 50ml of a solution containing 240mg Dobutamine.

Stage 2: Check that this is safe to give at the rate prescribed.

The prescription is for delivery to be 5ml/hour.

How much Dobutamine is this per minute?

If we have 240mg in 50ml.

There will be 24mg in 5ml of this solution.

24mg delivered over 60 minutes means $\frac{24}{60} = \frac{2}{5}$ or 0·4mg per minute

0·4mg = 400 microgram

The prescribed rate of 5ml/hour will deliver 400 microgram/minute.

◆ *Check* that this will deliver the required amount of 5 microgram/kg/min.

At weight 80kg, 5 microgram/kg = 400 microgram

Hence, the prescription is safe to give.

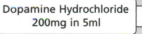

Practice exercise 8.4 Complex prescription involving inotropes

Follow the stages above to calculate and check the prescription below.

Mrs Vane, weight 53kg, requires inotropic support at a rate of 3 microgram/kg/min.

Name of drug	Amount	Route	Frequency
DOPAMINE	Solution made up as 3mg/kg in total volume of 50ml glucose 5%	IV via central line	3ml/hr

Label on ampoule:

> Dopamine Hydrochloride
> 200mg in 5ml

Recommended range to increase cardiac output is 2–10 microgram/kg/min.

Calculate correct to one decimal place;

1 Amount and volume of drug required to make up solution.

2 Volume of diluent.

3 Resulting delivery rate mg/hour.

4 Delivery rate in microgram/min.

Check your answers in Appendix E.

Nomograms

As we have seen, the calculations involved in inotropic doses and rate of administration can be quite complicated. To reduce the chance of error, many adult high dependency and intensive care units use **nomograms** or nomogram conversion charts to make certain frequently needed calculations easier for the medical and nursing staff. They are less common for children's nursing because of the small amounts used and the huge range of sizes among children.

Nomograms are complicated graphs which are usually converted to tables for use with drugs which are given by infusion on a microgram/ kilogram/minute (mcg/kg/min) basis. These are typically vasoactive or cardiac drugs such as dobutamine, dopamine, adrenaline, nor-adrenaline (all inotropes); and glyceryl trinitrate, which acts as a vasodilator.

We will use nomograms for Dopamine to show how they can be constructed in two main ways:

Method 1: The dose of dopamine is diluted into a *variable* volume of diluent (usually 0·9% saline) so that 1mcg/kg/min is achieved by setting the syringe pump at 1ml/hour.

Method 2: The dose of dopamine is diluted into a *fixed* volume of diluent and the syringe pump rate adjusted to give the appropriate mcg/kg/min.

Worked example 8.8 Dopamine nomogram method 1

The dose of Dopamine is diluted into a *variable* volume of diluent, so that 1mcg/kg/min is achieved by setting the syringe pump at 1ml/hour:

◆ The patient weighs 70kg. To achieve 1mcg/kg/min, we need to deliver 70 (70 × 1) mcg per minute.

◆ The syringe pump setting allows for ml per hour, so we need to convert our minutes to hours by multiplying by 60.

◆ 70mcg per minute will be 70 × 60 mcg per hour, or 4200mcg/hr.

Just take a minute to check that this is sensible.

For 1mcg/kg/min to equal 1ml/hr, the concentration of Dopamine needs to be 4200mcg per ml.

Label on ampoule:　　Dopamine Hydrochloride
200mg in 5ml

Dopamine is supplied as 200mg in 5ml, but remember that we need micrograms, so first let's change 200mg into micrograms (mcg):

1mg = 1000mcg

200mg = 200,000mcg

and so, the 5ml ampoule contains 200,000mcg of Dopamine.

What volume of diluent (v) do we need to dilute this to 4200mcg/ml? In other words, in what volume will 200,000mcg equal 4200mcg in 1ml?

Set up the equation:

$$\frac{200,000}{v} = \frac{4200}{1}$$

By dividing both sides by 4200 and multiplying both sides by v, we get:

$$\frac{200,000}{4200} = v$$

Simplify by dividing both top and bottom by 200 to get:

$$v = \frac{1000}{21} = 47{\cdot}6$$

125

Rounded to the nearest whole number, the volume we need is 48ml. This means we have to dilute the Dopamine to 48ml of solution to give 4200mcg of Dopamine per ml. As Dopamine is supplied in 5ml ampoules, we need (48–5) or 43ml of diluent.

As you can appreciate, this is a complex calculation and it would be tedious to have to do it for each patient. Therefore, in most intensive care environments, tabulations of nomograms like the one shown in Figure 8.1 are available.

In practice, the chart would have weight increasing in 1kg intervals. Using this table to prepare the solution means that a rate of 2ml/hr

mcg/kg/min	Patient's weight (kg)	Dopamine dose (mg)	Dopamine volume (ml)	Diluent volume (ml)	Total volume (ml)	Pump rate ml/hour
1	50	200	5	62	67	1
1	60	200	5	51	56	1
1	70	200	5	43	48	1
1	80	200	5	37	42	1
1	90	200	5	32	37	1

Figure 8.1 Extract from tabulated nomogram for Dopamine (method 1)

will deliver 2mcg/kg/min and 3ml/hr will deliver 3mcg/kg/min, and so on.

Note that for a patient of 50kg, the total volume exceeds the 60ml capacity of the syringes normally used in syringe pumps/drivers. In this case it is considered good practice to halve both the amount of dopamine and the total volume, resulting in 100mg Dopamine (2·5ml) diluted in 31ml of diluent to a total volume of 33·5ml.

Worked example 8.9 Dopamine nomogram method 2

The dose of Dopamine is diluted into a *fixed* volume of diluent and the syringe pump rate adjusted to give the appropriate mcg/kg/min:

◆ A 5ml ampoule of Dopamine contains 200mg. This is diluted with 45ml of diluent to a constant volume of 50ml.

◆ The concentration of Dopamine is now $\frac{200}{50}$ or 4mg/ml.

◆ 4mg = 4000mcg and so this is equivalent to 4000mcg/ml.

Using this solution, at what rate will we need to set the syringe pump/driver to deliver 1mcg/kg/min to a 70kg person?

1mcg/kg/min for a 70kg person = 70mcg/min or 70 × 60 mcg/hr = 4200mcg/hr

If the concentration is 4000mcg/ml, what rate must the pump be set at?

◆ *Estimate* we need just over 4000mcg per hour, so the rate of delivery should be just over 1ml per hour.

◆ *Calculate*. The calculation may be best explained by going back to one of the methods suggested for straightforward drug dosage calculations and finding what rate in ml/hr is equivalent to 1mcg/hour so that we can then multiply up to 4200mcg/hr.

We know that 1ml/hour = 4000mcg per hour

therefore $\frac{1}{4000}$ml/hr = 1mcg/hr

so $\frac{1}{4000}$ × 4200ml/hr = 4200mcg/hr

simplified, this becomes $\frac{42}{40}$ml/hr = 4200mcg/hr

or 1·05ml/hr will deliver 4200mcg/hr

Hence, the pump should be set at 1·05ml/hr.

Patient's weight (kg)	mcg/kg/min	Dopamine dose (mg)	Dopamine volume (ml)	Diluent volume (ml)	Total volume (ml)	Pump rate ml/hour
50	1	200	5	45	50	0·75
	2	200	5	45	50	1·5
	4	200	5	45	50	3·0
60	1	200	5	45	50	0·9
	2	200	5	45	50	1·8
	4	200	5	45	50	3·6
70	1	200	5	45	50	1·05
	2	200	5	45	50	2·1
	4	200	5	45	50	4·2
80	1	200	5	45	50	1·2
	2	200	5	45	50	2·4
	4	200	5	45	50	4·8

Figure 8.2 Extract from tabulated nomogram for Dopamine (method 2)

◆ *Check against the estimate* – just over 1ml/hr was our estimate.

As with method 1, repetitive calculations of this type can be tedious and the complicated nature of the calculation means that errors are more likely to be made. Hence a tabulated nomogram like the one in Figure 8.2 is very useful and also allows for higher doses of Dopamine to be calculated.

Neonates and paediatric intensive care

In high dependency areas such as Paediatric Intensive Care Units (PICU), children may be given continuous infusions of a variety of drugs via syringe drivers. Accurate calculations and checking regarding all aspects of the prescription and delivery are vitally important and this is one of the things a nurse will do when taking over the care of a child from another at the change of shift as well as when a prescription is new, or the syringe requires changing. You must be certain that you agree with the set-up which you are 'inheriting' as the accountability for the child's care passes to you at this point. Nomograms are not normally used in children's units and so calculation skills are vital.

Practice exercise 8.5 Using nomograms for giving inotropes

Work through the stages as illustrated above to prepare and check the following prescription using BOTH methods given by the Dopamine nomograms: (you will get two sets of answers).

Arnold Bennett weighs 60kg and is prescribed inotropic support.

Name of drug	Amount	Route	Dose	Frequency
DOPAMINE	200mg diluted to 50ml	IV via central line	4mcg/kg/min	continuous infusion

Label on ampoule:

> Dopamine 200mg
> in 5ml

Recommended adult dose is 2 microgram/kg/min – 5 microgram/kg/min.

1 Is this prescription suitable for the Dopamine nomogram?
2 How much diluent is required?
3 How much Dopamine will 1ml/hour deliver in mcg per minute? Give your answer correct to one decimal place.
4 What rate must the pump be set to deliver this prescription?

Check your answers in Appendix E.

Worked example 8.10 Inotropes in children

A newborn baby (3kg) who has had surgery to correct a congenital heart defect requires inotropic support in the form of a continuous infusion.

Name of drug	Amount	Route	Frequency
DOBUTAMINE	Solution made up as 90mg in total volume of 50ml	IV	1ml/hr

Label on ampoule:

> Dobutamine 50mg/ml

The recommended diluent is 5% glucose for dilution to a concentration of not more than 5mg/ml.

Recommended dosage for a newborn baby is 2–10 microgram/kg/min

This calculation is going to have several stages, but let's stick to the principles we have used throughout the book. We can use these first to calculate how to make up the prescribed solution.

◆ *Extract* the relevant information from the prescription:

Drug = 90mg Dobutamine

The diluent (50% glucose – but already made up as such, therefore the 50% is just a part of the labelling and does not come into the calculation). Made up to 50ml means we will need 50ml of diluent MINUS the volume of Dobutamine.

◆ *Check the prescription* – we'll leave this until we have calculated how to produce the required solution.

◆ *Check* that the drug is available in the same units as the prescription:

Yes, both are milligrams.

◆ *Estimate* an approximate answer:

We need 90mg and the drug is available as 50mg/ml and so we can estimate an amount of more than 1ml but less than 2ml.

◆ *Calculate*

Apply the formula: $\dfrac{what\ you\ want}{what\ you've\ got} \times what\ it's\ in = dose$

Substitute the known values to get your answer:

$\dfrac{90}{50} \times 1 = 1\cdot8ml$

◆ *Check this answer* against your approximation:

We had estimated more than 1ml and less than 2, so this is a sensible answer to have got.

The final step to preparing the solution is to look at the dilution instructions, which were:

Solution made up as 90mg in total volume of 50ml.

We need 1·8ml (90mg) of the drug to be made up to a total volume of 50ml and so we require:

(50 – 1·8)ml of diluent

= 48·2ml

Therefore, to make up the 50ml of solution to be infused, we need 1·8ml of Dobutamine in 48·2ml of 5% glucose.

◆ *Check that this is safe for our patient*:

Would this dose be right for a newborn baby?

The recommended dose is 2–10 microgram/kg/min.

We need to work this through as a separate calculation.

◆ *Check* that the drug is available in the same units as the prescription:

NO: the drug is available in mg/ml and we are looking at a recommended rate involving micrograms.

To work out whether the prescription fits with the recommended dose and rate for a newborn, we need to calculate:

◆ how many micrograms are contained in 1ml of the solution prescribed

◆ how many micrograms of drug is right for this weight of baby at the rate prescribed.

We have made up a solution of 90mg Dobutamine in 50ml, so what would that be in 1ml?

If 50ml = 90mg

Then $1\text{ml} = \dfrac{90}{50}\text{mg}$

To change this to microgram, multiply by 1000:

$$\dfrac{90}{50} \times 1000 = 90 \times 20$$

$$= 1800 \text{ microgram}$$

So, we have a solution which contains 1800 micrograms per ml.

Delivery rate = 1ml/hour which is what we will set the syringe driver to deliver and this will give the baby 1800 microgram of Dobutamine per hour. Is this a safe amount for the baby?

Recommended amount is 2–10 microgram/kg/min

We still need to calculate the rate of delivery in minutes to be able to compare it with the recommended dose:

1800 microgram per hour is how many microgram per minute?

◆ *Estimate or use a common-sense check*. Would the amount delivered in a minute be more or less than that delivered in an hour? The answer is, of course, less. So we need to divide by 60 to change the rate from hourly to per minute:

1800 microgram per hour = $\dfrac{1800}{60}$ mcg per minute

= 30 microgram per minute

Is this a safe amount for the baby? Remember, the recommended amount is 2–10 microgram/kg/min. The baby weighs 3kg, so the maximum amount for him would be 10×3 microgram per minute:

= 30 microgram per minute

This is exactly what we have calculated as being the amount delivered by the prescription and so we can safely go ahead with the delivery as instructed.

Practice exercise 8.6 Paediatric doses in intensive care

Paul, aged 12, weighs 37kg. He is on a ventilator and requires continuous sedation.

Name of drug	Dose/amount	Route	Frequency/time
MIDAZOLAM	40mg in 40ml	IV	3ml/hour

Label on ampoule:

Midazolam 10mg
in 2ml

The recommended diluent is 5% glucose. For sedation in intensive care for child over 6 months 60–120 microgram/kg/hour.

1 What volume of the drug illustrated is required to make up the prescription?

2 How much diluent is required?

3 What dose in micrograms per hour will he get?

4 What is the recommended range for a child of Paul's weight?

5 Is this safe to give?

Check your answers in Appendix E.

Calculations based on body surface area (BSA)

In children who are either extremely underweight or overweight for their age, dose by weight can be an unreliable method of calculating a therapeutic dose. Body surface area (BSA) gives a more accurate basis for calculating doses as it is a better indicator of metabolic processes. BSAs are calculated through use of standard tables, nomograms or by the use of a formula which provides an estimate of BSA based on the weight of the child (Table 8.1).

Table 8.1 Formula for BSA estimation

Weight range	Formula for estimation of BSA
1–5 kg	M^2 BSA = (0·05 × kg wt) + 0·05
6–10 kg	M^2 BSA = (0·04 × kg wt) + 0·10
11–20 kg	M^2 BSA = (0·03 × kg wt) + 0·20
21–70 kg	M^2 BSA = (0·02 × kg wt) + 0·40

Source: Rudolph, AM (1982) *Paediatrics*, 17th edn, Norwalk, CT: Appleton-Century-Crofts.

A table based on ideal body weights of children from newborn (full term) to 12 years is provided in the back of the BNF (March 2007), which also includes a formula for calculating paediatric doses. This formula is based on the assumption that the BSA of a 70kg adult is 1·8m^2 and looks like this:

$$\text{Approximate dose} = \frac{\text{BSA of child (m}^2)}{1\cdot8\text{m}^2} \times \text{Adult dose}$$

Thus, starting with an adult dose of 125mg, find the dose for a child with a BSA of 0·62m^2.

◆ *Applying the formula*

$$\text{Approximate dose} = \frac{0\cdot62}{1\cdot8} \times 125\text{mg}$$

◆ *Estimate* an answer by looking at the numbers and rounding where sensible:

$$\frac{0\cdot6}{1\cdot8} = \frac{6}{18} = \frac{1}{3}$$

one-third of 123 or ($\frac{1}{3} \times 123$) = 41

so we can estimate that the answer should be around 41mg. The actual calculation gives us 43mg.

As BSA is not commonly used by nurses for calculating medication dosage, there are no practice exercises for this section.

This is the final section of the book and if you have reached this point by systematically working through, you should be feeling more confident about using numbers in healthcare practice. We can all make mistakes but if you follow the process used throughout this book and check your answers against an estimate, you are more likely to be a safe practitioner when it comes to using numbers.

Appendix A
Some Common Abbreviations Used in Healthcare Practice

Abbreviation		Term in full	Definition, common examples of use and notes
weight	g	gram	Measure of mass – drug dosages
	kg	kilogram	Base unit for mass = 1000 grams – weight of individuals
	mg	milligram	One thousandth of a gram – drug dosages
	µg	microgram	One millionth of a gram – drug dosages. Use *not recommended* because of similarity to mg. Write in full
Vol	cl	centilitre	One hundredth of a litre
	L	litre	Base unit of volume. Note similarity to the number 1 and use with care
	mL or ml	millilitre	One thousandth of a litre – liquid feeds, medication, drainage, urine and intravenous fluids
	vol	volume	Measure of capacity
length	cm	centimetre	One hundredth of a metre – baby's length and head circumference, Central venous pressure (cm of water (H_2O))
	km	kilometre	One thousand metres – geographical distances
	m	metre	Base unit of length – height of individuals
	mm	millimetre	One thousandth of a metre – blood pressure measurement (mm of mercury (Hg))
	µm	micrometre	One millionth of a metre. Used in measurement of cell size

Abbreviation		Term in full	Definition, common examples of use and notes
Pressure	B/P	Blood Pressure	Measured in millimetres of mercury (mmHg)
	CVP	Central Venous Pressure	Usually measured in centimetres of water (cmH_2O)
	paO_2	Partial pressure of oxygen	Blood gas measurement
	Pa	Pascal	SI unit of pressure
Routes of administration	ID	Intradermal	Route of injection into the dermal layer
	IT	Intrathecal	Route of injection into the cerebro-spinal fluid within the dura
	IM	Intramuscular	Route of injection of drugs into the muscle
	IV	Intravenous	Route of administering fluid/drugs into a vein
	IVI	Intravenous infusion	Fluid given via a vein, sometimes shortened to IV
	O	Oral	By mouth
	SC	Subcutaneous	
Gases	CO_2	Carbon dioxide	
	H	Hydrogen	
	N	Nitrogen	
	NO_2	Nitrous oxide	
	O_2	Oxygen	
Prescription frequencies (May also be written in capitals)	a.c.	Ante cibum	Before food
	b.d.	Bis die	Twice daily
	o.d.	Omni die	Once a day
	o.m.	Omne mane	In the morning (sometimes written *mané*)
	o.n.	Omne nocte	At night (sometimes written *nocté*)
	p.c.	Post cibum	After food
	p.r.n.	Pro re nata	As required
	q.d.s.	Quater die sumendum	Four times per day

Abbreviation		Term in full	Definition, common examples of use and notes
	q.i.d.	Quater in die	Four times a day
	q.q.h.	Quaque quarta hora	Every four hours
	Stat.	Statim	Immediately
	t.d.s.	Ter die sumendum	Three times a day
	t.i.d.	Ter in die	Three times a day

Other abbreviations

£	pound (money)	
BNF	British National Formulary	
BSA	body surface area	Estimates of BSA may be more accurate than weight for calculating children's doses
cap.	capsule	
e/c	enteric coated	
FBC	fluid balance chart	
Hg	mercury	
H₂O	water	
hr	hour	
J	Joule	SI Unit of energy – used in defibrillation
lb	pound (weight)	
min	minute	
NMC	Nursing and Midwifery Council	Statutory regulatory body for nurses and midwives in UK
oz	ounce	
PICU	Paediatric intensive care unit	
POM	Prescription only medicine	
SI	Système International d'Unités	International System of units – metric
Tab.	tablet	

Appendix B
Mathematical symbols

Symbol	Meaning
+	plus
−	minus
±	plus or minus
×	multiplied by
*	
÷	divided by
/	
=	equals
≈	approximately equal to
%	percent
∴	therefore
:	ratio of
>	greater than
<	less than
≤	less than or equal to
≥	more than or equal to

Appendix C
Glossary

Addition	The process of putting numbers together or combining them to find their *sum*.
Bolus	An amount given in one go. A one-off dose.
Centile	Centile charts show the distribution of a parameter within the population.
Decimal fraction	The proper name for decimals.
Denominator	The number below the line in a fraction.
Dialysis	Process by which blood is filtered to remove impurities.
Digit	Any number from 0 to 9.
Diluent or Dilutent	A liquid used to reconstitute a powder to produce a solution or a liquid used to dilute another to produce a weaker solution.
Displacement value	The increase in volume of a diluent when mixed with a powder.
Division	The process of separating an amount into an equal number of parts. The result is the *quotient*.
Dose/dosage	The amount of drug prescribed.
Dyscalculia	Number dyslexia.
Dyslexia	Learning disability which causes a range of difficulties in reading and writing.
Enteric coated	Tablets with a special coating to protect the stomach lining.
Epidural	Refers to injection/infusion into the epidural space.

Equation   A statement of equality between two things.

Fraction   Part of a whole number, e.g. $\frac{3}{4}$.

Imperial measure   Measures used prior to decimalization, e.g. pounds and ounces.

Intrathecal   Into the cerebro-spinal fluid within the dura.

Mixed number   A whole number and a fraction, e.g. $3\frac{1}{2}$.

Multiplication   Repeated addition. The number is added to itself a specific number of times resulting in the *product*.

Nomogram   A graphical representation of an equation.

Numerator   The number above the line in a fraction.

Reconstitution   Making up a solution by combining powder with a diluent.

Solute   Substance which dissolves.

Subtraction   The opposite of addition, resulting in their *difference*.

Top-heavy fraction   Fraction in which the numerator is greater than the denominator. May be changed to a mixed number.

See also Appendix A for abbreviations.

Appendix D
Answers to Self-Assessment

1	15,034	**16**	$11\frac{1}{5}$	**30**	90%
2	1,206,907	**17**	£2.25	**31**	80%
3	1553	**18**	£30.25	**32**	0·25
4	7437	**19**	36·374	**33**	1·7
5	1275	**20**	162·2	**34**	0·25
6	986	**21**	42·98	**35**	0·8
7	858	**22**	1125	**36**	$\frac{3}{4}$
8	17,406	**23**	3·5	**37**	$\frac{1}{20}$
9	171	**24**	8·25	**38**	$\frac{1}{5}$
10	302	**25**	17·4	**39**	$\frac{1}{25}$
11	$\frac{1}{4}$	**26**	2·55	**40**	0·5gram
12	$\frac{1}{3}$	**27**	0·555	**41**	250mg
13	$2\frac{11}{20}$	**28**	75%	**42**	0·1 litre
14	$2\frac{1}{2}$	**29**	2·5%	**43**	2000 micrograms
15	$31\frac{1}{4}$				

Appendix E
Answers to Practice Exercises

1.1 Whole numbers

1 1,234,567
2 5,300,050
3 25,007
4 112,600
5 8,004

1.2 Rounding decimals

1 245·4
2 12·1
3 30·1
4 8·6
5 13·29
6 0·3
7 50·9
8 1·85
9 100
10 7

1.3 Fractions

1 $\frac{5}{10}$

2 $10\frac{7}{10}$

3 $1\frac{6}{100}$

4 $\frac{35}{100}$

5 $\frac{109}{1000}$

2.1 Multiplication of whole numbers

1 42 tablets

2 120ml

3 276 hours

2.2 Division of whole numbers

1 150mg

2 200ml

3 65 per ward and 5 over

4 £150

2.3 Addition and subtraction of decimals

1 78·4

2 54·5

3 25·775

4 84·45

5 274·35

2.4 Multiplying decimals

1 27·5

2 1250

3 414·84

4 681·6

5 15

2.5 Dividing decimals

1 0·825

2 0·0102

3 26·7

4 23

5 25

2.6 Changing decimals to fractions and fractions to decimals

1 40·25

2 $\frac{2}{5}$

3 $2\frac{1}{3}$

4 $\frac{1}{8}$

5 0·64

6 $\frac{3}{4}$

7 0·75

2.7 Addition and subtraction of fractions

1 $\frac{9}{8} = 1\frac{1}{8}$

2 $\frac{1}{12}$

3 $\frac{7}{6} = 1\frac{1}{6}$

4 $\frac{14}{24} = \frac{7}{12}$

2.8 Multiplying and dividing fractions

1 $\frac{3}{20}$

2 $\frac{3}{10}$

3 $\frac{1}{5}$

4 $\frac{3}{8}$

5 $1\frac{1}{4}$

2.9 Solving simple equations

1 $r = 166·7$

2 $t = 4$

3 $v = 1000$

3.1 Money management

1   £14.22

2   £13.38

3   £12.88

4 £112.10

5 £123.98

3.2 Time

1 $6\frac{1}{2}$ hrs
2 01.40 hrs
3 06.30 hrs
4 12.15 hrs
5 16.49 hrs

3.3 Metric conversion

1 250mg
2 7·5mg
3 1300ml
4 25 nanogram
5 1·25g

3.4 Conversion of imperial to metric measures and vice versa (i)

1 6lb 15oz
2 19 inches
3 0·2kg
4 5·6oz
5 3·2oz

3.5 Conversion of imperial to metric measures and vice versa (ii)

1 4 stone 2lb
2 3 ft 9 inches
3 6 stone 4lb
4 12 inches

3.6 Conversion of imperial to metric measures and vice versa (iii)

1 75·5kg
2 167cm
3 8lb
4 11 stone 4lb

3.7 Growth charts (i)

1 90th

2 50th

3 About 80cm

3.8 Symphysis-fundal height chart

1 90th

2 37cm

3 Being on the 90th centile means that for every 100 women at this stage in pregnancy, 10 are likely to have a fundus higher than this and 90 will be lower.

3.9 Growth charts (ii)

1 Just below the 5th centile

2 Yes

3 Timmy is definitely smaller than average, but not necessarily abnormal. Being on this centile means that for every 100 boys of his age, 96 will be taller and heavier than Timmy.

3.10 Growth charts (iii)

1 5th centile for height

2 95th centile for weight

3 This indicates that although both measurements are within the normal range for a 17-year-old boy, John would be considered overweight for his height.

4.1 Multiple unit drug calculations

1 2 tablets

2 2 tablets

3 3 tablets

4 2 tablets

4.2 Sub-unit drug calculations

1 $\frac{1}{2}$ tablet

2 $1\frac{1}{2}$ tablets

3 $\frac{1}{2}$ tablet

4.3 Tablets and capsules drug calculations (i)

1 2 capsules

2 1 tablet

3 3 tablets

4 2 tablets

5 2 capsules

6 $\frac{1}{2}$ tablet

4.4 Tablets and capsules drug calculations (ii)

1 10 tablets

2 2 tablets

3 1 capsule

4 2 tablets

5.1 Oral liquid medication

1 15ml

2 7·5ml

3 7·5ml

4 2ml

5.2 Oral liquid medications with prescription check

1 Yes, prescription is within recommended range, 8·3ml is required.

2 Yes, prescription is within recommended range, 2·5ml is required.

3 Yes, prescription is within recommended range, 5ml is required.

4 Yes, prescription is within recommended range, 10ml is required.

5.3 Weight-based prescriptions (adults)

1 3060 microgram or 3mg
2 Yes, it is the correct dose for her weight and below the daily maximum.
3 $1\frac{1}{2}$ tablets
4 $1\frac{1}{2}$ tablets
5 15ml
6 $\frac{1}{2}$ tablet

5.4 Weight-based prescriptions (children)

1 Yes, the prescription is within the recommended dose range for weight. Give 4ml.
2 Yes, the prescription is within the recommended dose range for weight. Give 3ml.
3 Yes, the prescription is within the recommended dose range for weight. Give 8·3ml.

5.5 Drug calculations

1 5ml
2 10ml
3 6ml
4 Yes, the prescription is within the recommended dose range for a child of this age and weight. Give 8·75ml.

6.1 Injections

1 3ml
2 0·6ml
3 1·5ml
4 2ml

6.2 Reconstitution of powdered preparations

1 Prescription check – 400mg 8 hourly = 1200mg daily.
Recommended dose for weight 800–1600mg daily.
Give 2·3ml
2 21ml

6.3 Intravenous rates of infusion, volumetric pumps (ml/hr)

1   167ml/hr
2   142·9ml/hr
3   250ml/hr
4   83·3ml/hr
5   125ml/hr
6   133·3ml/hr

6.4 Manual IV drip rates

1   33 drops per minute
2   25 drops per minute
3   28 drops per minute
4   42 drops per minute
5   28 drops per minute
6   67 drops per minute

6.5 Syringe drivers

1   Prescription check – 2mg/kg = 50mg
    To give 62·5ml over 30 mins (every 8 hours)
    set syringe driver at 125ml/hr.
2   1·5ml over 24 hours

7.1 Fluid balance chart (i)

1   Total input = 3260ml
2   Total output = 2920ml
3   24-hour balance = +340ml

7.2 Fluid balance chart (ii)

1   3990ml
2   3850ml
3   +140ml
4   1850ml

7.3 Peritoneal dialysis record

1 −55ml
2 +0·02kg

7.4 Infant feeds

1 361·5ml, 30ml per feed
2 622·5ml, 104ml per feed
3 564ml, 71ml per feed

7.5 High dependency Infant fluids

1 288ml
2 84ml
3 35·2ml
4 169ml
5 115·2ml
6 24ml
7 44ml
8 47·2ml
9 172·8ml
10 104·8ml
11 19·2ml
12 268·8ml

8.1 Percentages

1 40%
2 6%
3 80%
4 1%
5 0·7
6 0·125
7 21
8 50

9 20g

10 5mg/ml

11 3·1%

12 33·3%

8.2 Ratio and proportions

1 2%

2 1 in 10,000

3 0·05%

4 1 in 200

5 0·02%

8.3 Percentage and proportions

1 1mg

2 5ml of 10% solution and 45ml diluent

3 24ml Bupivacaine 0·25% and 36ml diluent

4 0·8mg or 800 micrograms

8.4 Complex prescription involving inotropes

1 159mg or 4ml

2 46ml diluent

3 9·5mg/hour

4 159 microgram/min

8.5 Using nomograms for giving inotropes

	Method 1	Method 2
1	Yes	Yes
2	51ml	45ml
3	59·5mcg	66·7mcg
4	4ml/hr	3·6ml/hr

8.6 Paediatric doses in intensive care

1 8ml

2 32ml

3 3000 micrograms

4 2220–4440 microgram/hour

5 Yes, this is within the recommended range